FIRE SAFETY AWARENESS FOR VEHICLE DRIVERS
A STEP-BY-STEP GUIDE

Blessing Isaackson

Disclaimer

This publication is intended for educational and informational purposes only. The content is based on current best practices, legislation, and guidance available at the time of publication. It does not constitute legal, technical, or professional advice, and should not be relied upon as a substitute for formal fire safety training or consultation with qualified professionals.

While every effort has been made to ensure the accuracy of the information provided, the author and publisher accept no responsibility or liability for any loss, damage, injury, or consequence arising from the use or misuse of this guide. Readers are advised to refer to current legislation, professional training providers, and employer policies for specific requirements related to fire safety and vehicle operation.

Laws, regulations, and safety standards may change over time. It is the responsibility of the reader, driver, or employer to remain informed of and compliant with all applicable fire safety laws and driving regulations relevant to their jurisdiction and vehicle type.

Use of this guide is at your own discretion and risk.

FIRE SAFETY AWARENESS FOR VEHICLE DRIVERS: A STEP-BY-STEP GUIDE
© Blessing Isaackson, [2025]
All rights reserved.

No part of this publication may be copied, reproduced, stored in a retrieval system, transmitted in any form or by any means—electronic, mechanical, photocopying, recording, scanning, or otherwise—without the prior written permission of the author, except as permitted by UK copyright law under the Copyright, Designs and Patents Act 1988.

This book is intended solely for personal or educational use. Any unauthorised use—including but not limited to commercial distribution, adaptation, or sale—is strictly prohibited and may result in legal action.

The author asserts their moral right to be identified as the author of this work. ("Robin Hobb asserts the moral right to be identified as the author of ...")

For permission requests, contact:
Blessing Isaackson
info@firstaidtutors.co.uk

ISBN: 978-1-0683557-9-0

Table of Contents

INTRODUCTION 1
About the Author 3
The purpose of this book 4
WHAT IS FIRE? 7
WHY FIRE SAFETY MATTERS FOR DRIVERS 8
Dealing with an Emergency Fire in a Vehicle on the Motorway 10
KEY FIRE SAFETY PRACTICES FOR DRIVERS 13
WHAT TO DO IN THE CASE OF A VEHICLE FIRE 14
CONSEQUENCES OF FIRE: HEAT, SMOKE, AND TOXIC GASES 15
HIGH-RISK FIRE ENVIRONMENTS FOR VEHICLES 17
DRIVER AWARENESS TIPS 21
Vehicle Fires in the UK 23
Regional & Urban Insights 25
⚡ Electric Vehicle & Lithium-Ion Battery Fires 25
Fire Detection and Suppression Systems in Vehicles 26
Maintenance and Inspection 28
Legal and Regulatory Considerations (UK) 29
Key Takeaways 29
Know Your Fire Extinguisher 30
PASS Technique for Using a Fire Extinguisher 31
Safe Usage Tips 31
Legal and Practical Considerations (UK) 32
Safe Handling of Flammable Liquids and Materials in Vehicles 33
Safe Storage in the Vehicle 34
WHAT TO AVOID 35
Fire Safety Responsibilities of Employed Drivers 37
Summary of Legal Responsibilities 38
Vehicle Fire Safety Checklist (Daily Use) 39

Post-Incident Checklist for Drivers 40

Vehicle Fires in the UK: Intentional Fires – Arson, Fraud, and Criminal Cover-up 41

Responsibilities of Employers under UK Fire Safety Law 46

Responsibilities of Employees under UK Fire Safety Law 55

Electrical Fires: Key Hazards 63

Fire Safety Compliance Essentials (UK) 69

Causes of Motor Vehicle Fires 70

Classes of Fire (UK Classification – BS EN 2:1992) 75

Class A – Solid Combustible Materials 75

Class B – Flammable Liquids 76

Class C – Flammable Gases 77

Class D – Combustible Metals 78

Class F – Cooking Oils and Fats 81

Fire Extinguisher Types & Their Uses 82

Best Fire Extinguishers for Vehicles (UK Guide) 90

Best Practice by Vehicle Type 96

Electric Vehicles 104

Vehicles Legally Required to Carry Fire Extinguishers (UK) 107

General Safety & Maintenance Requirements 109

Recommended Types of Extinguishers for Vehicles 110

Fire Safety Rules for Company Cars (UK Guidance) 111

ADR & CDG Regulations: Fire Extinguisher Requirements for Vehicles Carrying Dangerous Goods 114

Which Vehicles Must Comply? 114

ADR Fire Extinguisher Requirements by Vehicle Weight 115

Fire Extinguisher Maintenance Requirements 117

⚠ Non-Compliance Risks 117

Common Causes of Vehicle Fires 118

AFFF FIRE EXTINGUISERS 121

What Are AFFF Fire Extinguishers? 122

Legal Framework: Regulatory Reform (Fire Safety) Order 2005 130
Fire Safety Responsibilities of Employers 131
Fire Safety Responsibilities of Employed Drivers 133
RISK ASSESSMENT **139**
APPENDICES **145**
Appendix A: vehicle Driver Risk assessment Template 145
Appendix B: Fire Safety Training Record Template 150
APPENDIX C: Fire Extinguisher User Guide for Vehicle Drivers 153
APPENDIX D LEGAL REFERENCE SUMMARY 156
Bibliography 159
Glossary & Resources 161

INTRODUCTION

FIRE SAFETY AWARENESS FOR VEHICLE DRIVERS: A STEP-BY-STEP GUIDE

by **Blessing Isaackson**

Every year in the United Kingdom, thousands of vehicle fires are reported, many of which could have been prevented or safely managed with the proper knowledge and preparation. Fires involving vehicles not only pose a serious risk to drivers, passengers, and the public, but they also cause significant disruption and financial loss. Whether caused by mechanical failure, human error, or deliberate acts, the consequences can be devastating.

Fire Safety Awareness for Vehicle Drivers: A Step-by-Step Guide has been written to empower drivers with the practical knowledge and confidence needed to understand, prevent, and respond effectively to fire-related incidents involving vehicles. Drawing from up-to-date fire safety legislation, best practice guidance, and real-world examples, this guide provides essential information tailored specifically for vehicle operators—whether you're a commercial driver, fleet manager, or private motorist.

This book covers a wide range of topics, including:

- The science of fire and how it starts in vehicles
- "Common causes of vehicle fires and how to prevent them" ("Vehicle Fires: how they start, spread, and how to prevent them")

- Your legal responsibilities under current UK fire safety legislation
- Fire detection, suppression, and emergency response equipment
- Safe evacuation procedures and post-incident actions
- Realistic scenario-based training and checklists

By the end of this guide, you will have a thorough understanding of your role in fire safety as a vehicle driver, and the practical tools to protect yourself and others on the road. Fire safety is not just a legal obligation—it is a life-saving responsibility.

Stay informed. Stay prepared. Stay safe.

About the Author

Key Credentials at a Glance

Credential	Details
Role	Managing Director, Fairview Training Ltd, First Aid Tutors, Director of the Fire Marshal Academy
Specialisations	First aid training, medical emergencies, fire safety education
Author of	Manuals including *Fire Safety for Vehicle Drivers, First Aid, Immediate Life Support for Dentists, Managing Medical Emergencies in A Dental Practice, Dental Basic Life Support- A Step-By-Step Handbook*, and the *Fire Safety Manual*
Audience	Emergency preparedness teams, vehicle drivers, safety trainers, and healthcare staff
Style	Step-by-step, accessible, practice-oriented

Blessing Isaackson brings together theoretical knowledge, practical expertise, and structured training experience to make complex safety topics accessible to all. His guide on fire safety for vehicle drivers aims to significantly reduce risks by combining prevention strategies with clear action plans, helping both professional drivers and everyday motorists respond effectively in emergencies.

The purpose of this book

The purpose of this book is to equip vehicle drivers with essential knowledge and practical guidance on fire prevention, early detection, and appropriate emergency response in the event of a vehicle fire. Motor vehicle fires, though often overlooked, pose serious risks to life, property, and public safety. Many of these incidents are preventable through proper awareness, maintenance, and preparedness.
Practices for refuelling, carrying flammable materials, and managing electrical or mechanical systems. This step-by-step guide aims to:

1. **Raise Awareness** about the common causes and warning signs of vehicle fires.
2. **Educate Drivers** on how to inspect and maintain their vehicles to reduce fire risks.
3. **Promote Safe** faults.
4. **Provide Clear Instructions** on how to respond safely and effectively if a fire occurs, including evacuation, use of fire extinguishers, and alerting emergency services.
5. **Support Legal and Regulatory Compliance** by explaining relevant fire safety laws, insurance considerations, and driver responsibilities.

By enhancing fire safety awareness among drivers, this book seeks to reduce the incidence and impact of vehicle fires, safeguard lives, and promote a culture of safety and responsibility on the road.

Importance of Fire Safety for Drivers

Fire safety is a critical aspect of responsible driving that is often underestimated. Vehicle fires can occur suddenly and escalate rapidly, endangering the lives of drivers, passengers, other road users, and emergency responders. Understanding and practising fire safety is essential for several key reasons:

1. **Protecting Lives**

   Vehicle fires can lead to severe injuries or fatalities if not managed quickly and appropriately. Fire safety awareness enables drivers to act swiftly to evacuate occupants, use extinguishers if safe, and prevent loss of life.

2. **Preventing Property Damage**

   Motor vehicles are valuable assets. Fires can result in complete vehicle loss and potentially spread to nearby vehicles, structures, or roadside vegetation. Early detection and prevention measures can significantly reduce damage.

3. **Reducing Risk of Collisions**

   A vehicle fire or smoke inside the cabin can cause panic or distraction, leading to accidents. Understanding how to handle such emergencies helps maintain road safety for all users.

4. **Complying with Legal and Insurance Requirements**

   Many jurisdictions require that commercial drivers and transport companies adhere to fire safety regulations, including carrying fire extinguishers and conducting vehicle checks. Insurance claims may be denied if negligence in fire safety is proven.

5. **Minimising Environmental Impact**

   Vehicle fires release toxic gases and chemicals that pollute the air and soil. Preventing fires contributes to environmental protection and public health.

6. **Enhancing Public and Workplace Safety**

   For professional drivers, fire safety is not only a personal responsibility but also a workplace requirement. Protecting passengers, cargo, and infrastructure is essential for those in transport and logistics industries.

7. **Building Confidence and Preparedness**

   Drivers who are educated and prepared for fire-related emergencies are more confident and capable of making calm, informed decisions during high-pressure situations.

In summary, fire safety is not just a precaution—it is a fundamental part of safe driving that protects lives, property, and the environment.

WHAT IS FIRE?

Fire is the result of a **chemical reaction** known as **combustion**, which occurs when a fuel source reacts with oxygen in the presence of sufficient heat. This reaction releases **heat**, **light**, and often **smoke and toxic gases** such as carbon monoxide and hydrogen cyanide. The three essential elements for fire—**heat, fuel, and oxygen**—are represented in the **fire triangle**.

WHY FIRE SAFETY MATTERS FOR DRIVERS

1. **Vehicle Fires Can Be Deadly**
    - Vehicle fires can escalate rapidly due to flammable materials like fuel, oil, and electrical components.
    - Fires may cause explosions, toxic smoke inhalation, or severe burns.
2. **Electrical and Fuel Systems Are High-Risk Areas**
    - Modern vehicles have complex electrical systems and high-pressure fuel lines that can ignite easily if damaged.
    - Faulty wiring, battery malfunctions, or fuel leaks are common causes of fires.
3. **Fires Can Occur Without a Collision**
    - Overheated engines, electrical shorts, or mechanical failures can lead to spontaneous combustion even if the car hasn't been in a crash.
4. **Fire Can Trap Occupants**
    - Fires often disable electronic systems, including door locks and windows, making escape more difficult.
    - Immediate action and knowledge of escape protocols are vital.
5. **Legal and Financial Consequences**
    - Failure to maintain fire-safe vehicles may lead to insurance claim rejections or legal liabilities.

- Employers have a legal duty under UK health and safety law to ensure work vehicles are safe and fit for use.

Dealing with an Emergency Fire in a Vehicle on the Motorway

1. Stop Safely

- If your vehicle catches fire, **signal left and pull over** as soon as it is safe:
    - Use the **hard shoulder** or an **emergency refuge area** (on smart motorways).
    - If that's not possible, **stop as far to the left as you can**, keeping clear of traffic.
- **Turn wheels left** and **switch on hazard lights**.
- **Do not remain in the vehicle.**

Highway Code Rule 275 & 277

2. Switch Off & Exit Immediately

- Turn off the engine and **remove the key**.
- Exit the vehicle quickly and **leave all belongings behind**.
- Where possible, exit using the **left-hand (non-traffic side) doors**.

Rule 277

3. Move to Safety

- Move **behind a safety barrier**, away from traffic.
- If safe, position yourself **uphill and upwind** of the vehicle to avoid smoke or fumes.

- Never stand on the carriageway.

Rule 277

4. Call 999

- Dial **999** and ask for the **fire and rescue service**.
- Provide:
    - **Motorway name/number** (e.g., M25)
    - **Nearest junction** or **marker post number**
    - **Direction of travel** (e.g., northbound)
    - **Nature of the fire** (e.g., "engine fire")

Rule 277

5. Do Not Attempt to Extinguish the Fire If:

- Flames are coming from **inside the vehicle or engine bay**.
- You don't have a suitable extinguisher (**ABC dry powder**).
- You're **not trained or confident** to use it.

Use an extinguisher **only if all below apply**:

- The fire is **tiny and contained**.
- You have the **correct extinguisher**.
- You are trained, and it's **safe with an escape route**.

6. Warn Other Road Users – If Safe

- On **non-motorway roads**, place a **warning triangle** at least **45 metres (147 ft)** behind the vehicle.

- **Never use warning triangles on motorways**—they are prohibited.

Rule 277

7. Wait for Help

- **Do not return to the vehicle** under any circumstances.
- Stay behind a barrier until emergency services arrive.
- Let them know if you're carrying any **hazardous materials**.

Safety Notes (Legal & Practical)

Item	Advice
Fire extinguisher	Not legally required for private cars; **recommended** for commercial vehicles
High-vis vest	**Recommended**, especially at night
Stopping on motorways	Only in emergencies – **use hard shoulder or refuge areas**
Smart motorways	Use emergency refuge areas where available
Rules to follow	Highway Code Rules **275–283**

Recommended Kit to Carry

- ABC **dry powder fire extinguisher** (1–2 kg, car-rated)
- **High-visibility vest**
- **Warning triangle** (for use on non-motorways)
- **Fully charged mobile phone** + power bank
- **First aid kit**

KEY FIRE SAFETY PRACTICES FOR DRIVERS

- **Regular Maintenance**
    - Schedule vehicle inspections to identify fuel, oil, and electrical faults early.
    - Replace worn-out parts and fix leaks immediately.
- **Carry a Vehicle Fire Extinguisher**
    - Ensure it's suitable for Class B (flammable liquids) and Class C (electrical fires).
    - Know how to use it safely (PASS: Pull, Aim, Squeeze, Sweep).
- **Respond Quickly to Warning Signs**
    - Look for smoke, burning smells, warning lights, or engine overheating.
    - Stop the car safely, turn off the engine, and exit immediately if fire is suspected.
- **Don't Overload Electrical Systems**
    - Avoid using faulty chargers, overloaded power adapters, or makeshift electrical connections.
- **Keep Flammable Items Secure**
    - Store items like aerosols, fuel containers, or cleaning sprays away from heat sources.

WHAT TO DO IN THE CASE OF A VEHICLE FIRE

1. **Pull Over Safely**
    - Stop in a safe location away from traffic and structures.
2. **Turn Off Ignition**
    - This stops fuel flow and electrical power.
3. **Evacuate Immediately**
    - Ensure all passengers get out and move at least 100 feet away.
4. **Call Emergency Services**
    - Dial 999 and clearly state your location and situation.
5. **Do Not Open the Bonnet**
    - Introducing oxygen can intensify the fire.

Final Thoughts

Fire safety is not just for buildings—it is equally essential on the road. By maintaining your vehicle, recognising early warning signs, and knowing how to act during an emergency, you protect yourself, your passengers, and others around you.

Remember: Prevention, preparation, and quick action save lives.

CONSEQUENCES OF FIRE: HEAT, SMOKE, AND TOXIC GASES

Understanding the dangers associated with fire goes beyond just flames. The real and immediate threats come from **extreme heat, dense smoke**, and **toxic gases**—all of which can be fatal within moments, especially in the confined space of a vehicle.

1. Extreme Heat

- **Temperatures inside a vehicle fire** can quickly reach **600–1,100°C (1,100–2,000°F)**.
- This heat can cause:
    - Severe burns on contact.
    - Melting of vehicle parts and interior components (plastic, vinyl, etc.).
    - Explosion of pressurised items (fuel tanks, airbags, tyres).
- Even if a person is not directly in contact with flames, **radiant heat** can burn skin and damage the respiratory tract.

2. Smoke Inhalation

- Most fire-related deaths are not caused by burns but by **smoke inhalation**.
- Vehicle fires produce thick, dark smoke that:
    - Obscures vision, making it harder to escape or locate passengers.

- Causes **coughing, choking, disorientation**, and **loss of consciousness**.
- Irritates eyes, nose, and throat almost instantly.

☠ 3. Toxic Gases

- Burning materials (upholstery, plastics, wiring) release **highly toxic gases**, including:
    - **Carbon monoxide (CO):** Odourless, colourless gas that reduces oxygen to the brain and can lead to unconsciousness within minutes.
    - **Hydrogen cyanide (HCN):** Released from burning plastics and synthetic materials; affects cellular oxygen use and can be rapidly fatal.
    - **Phosgene and dioxins:** Formed by burning refrigerants or PVC; extremely harmful to lungs and nervous system.

Inhalation of these gases for even a few seconds can cause serious injury or death.

HIGH-RISK FIRE ENVIRONMENTS FOR VEHICLES

Certain environments and conditions significantly increase the risk of vehicle fires. Drivers must be especially alert and proactive when operating in or around these high-risk settings.

1. High-Traffic Urban Areas

- **Frequent stop-start driving** increases engine and brake wear, raising the risk of overheating.
- **Accidents and collisions** are more common, increasing the likelihood of fuel system damage or electrical fires.
- **Limited emergency access** may delay fire services, increasing danger.

2. Hot Weather and Heatwaves

- High ambient temperatures strain **cooling systems**, leading to overheating engines.
- **Fuel vapour pressure increases**, making fuel systems more volatile.
- Flammable materials (e.g. fuel, oil, tyres) are more susceptible to ignition.

3. Fuel Stations and Refuelling Areas

- **Open sources of fuel** (petrol, diesel, LPG) pose an obvious ignition risk.

- Static electricity, hot engines, or lit cigarettes can ignite vapours.
- Mobile phones or improper fuel handling may contribute to accidental fires.

4. Work Vehicles in Industrial or Construction Zones

- Exposure to **flammable chemicals**, solvents, paints, or gas cylinders.
- Accumulated dust, debris, and grease in engine compartments can catch fire.
- Vehicles may carry **welding equipment**, **batteries**, or **pressurised containers**.

5. Off-Road or Rural Areas

- **Dry vegetation**, leaves, or grass can catch fire from a hot exhaust or catalytic converter.
- **Limited access to emergency help** and **a lack of nearby water sources increase** severity.
- **Long travel distances** may delay recognition of mechanical issues like oil or coolant leaks.

6. Underground Car Parks and Tunnels

- Poor ventilation means **smoke and toxic gases** build up quickly in the event of fire.
- **Heat is trapped**, intensifying fire spread.
- Restricted space can make evacuation and emergency response difficult.

7. Vehicles with Modified or Damaged Electrical Systems

- Aftermarket modifications (e.g. subwoofers, lighting, chargers) may overload circuits.
- Poorly installed wiring can lead to **short circuits** or **sparks**. ("Common Fire Hazards in Commercial Buildings and How to Mitigate Them")
- Damaged battery terminals or improper jump-starting can start fires instantly.

8. Hybrid and Electric Vehicles

- High-voltage battery systems pose **unique fire risks**, especially if damaged.
- **Thermal runaway** in lithium-ion batteries can cause intense fires that are difficult to extinguish.
- Risk of delayed ignition—even after a crash or once power is cut off.

Summary Table: High-Risk Environments

Environment	Key Fire Risks
Urban traffic areas	Collisions, overheating, electrical overloads
Hot weather	Overheating, fuel vapour ignition
Fuel stations	Fuel vapours, static discharge, open flames
Industrial/construction zones	Flammable materials, work equipment

Environment	Key Fire Risks
Rural/off-road areas	Dry vegetation, engine debris, delayed response
Underground/tunnels	Smoke buildup, trapped heat, limited escape routes
Modified/damaged systems	Overloaded wiring, faulty batteries
Electric/hybrid vehicles	Battery fires, thermal runaway

DRIVER AWARENESS TIPS

- Conduct **daily vehicle checks**—look for leaks, exposed wires, or warning lights.
- **Avoid parking over dry grass or leaves** after driving.
- Never leave **running vehicles unattended** in high-risk areas.
- Report and repair **overheating issues or electrical faults** immediately.

Fire risk increases when awareness decreases. Knowing the environments where vehicle fires are more likely helps drivers stay alert, prepared, and safe.

Why This Matters for Drivers

- Vehicle occupants may have **less than 1 minute** to evacuate before conditions become lethal.
- The **build-up of smoke and gases** in a closed space (like a car or van) is far faster than in open-air fires.
- **Opening doors or windows during a fire** can worsen smoke flow or fuel the flames with fresh oxygen.

Key Safety Takeaways

- **Evacuate immediately** at the first sign of smoke or fire—don't attempt to retrieve belongings.
- **Stay low** if smoke is present air is clearer closer to the floor.
- **Never re-enter** a burning vehicle.
- Call **999** as soon as you are at a safe distance.

Summary

Danger	Effect on Occupants
Heat	Burns, equipment failure, explosion risk
Smoke	Disorientation, impaired vision, suffocation
Toxic Gases	Unconsciousness, poisoning, death

Act fast. Seconds matter. Fire doesn't wait—and neither should you.

Vehicle Fires in the UK

Vehicle fires are a significant concern for fire safety in the UK. According to government fire statistics:

- Over **100,000 vehicle fires** occur each year across the country—this means around **300 incidents every day**.
- Approximately **65% of these fires are intentional**, commonly set to:
    - Destroy evidence of other criminal activity (e.g., stolen vehicles).
    - Commit insurance fraud.
    - Engage in acts of vandalism or arson.
- Only **35% of vehicle fires are accidental**, typically caused by mechanical faults, electrical failures, overheating, or poor maintenance.

These figures underscore the importance of both fire prevention strategies and public awareness, particularly in high-risk environments such as commercial transportation, public service vehicles, and areas with a high incidence of crime.

Understanding the **nature, causes, and consequences of fire** is the first step in ensuring effective prevention, appropriate emergency response, and compliance with UK fire safety legislation.

Overall Vehicle Fires

- Approximately **100,000 vehicle fires per year**, averaging nearly 300 a day across the UK theguardian.com+15fireservice.co.uk+15housegrail.com+15.
- Between July 2022 and June 2023, **19,256 serious road vehicle fires** were reported housegrail.com+1reddit.com+1.

Accidental vs Deliberate Fires

- Around **60–65%** of vehicle fires are **deliberate**, often due to arson, insurance fraud, or criminal motives bbc.co.uk+7fireservice.co.uk+7autoexpress.co.uk+7.
- Conversely, **35–40%** stem from **accidental causes** such as mechanical or electrical faults acorninsure.co.uk.
- Notably, from 2019/20 to 2023/24, the proportion of **accidental fires increased to ~60%**, up from ~52% theguardian.com+5standard.co.uk+5independent.co.uk+5.

Trends Over Time

- Vehicle fire incidents decreased by ~14%: down from ~21,878 (2015–2020 average) to **18,906** in 2023/24 autoexpress.co.uk+4standard.co.uk+4independent.co.uk+4.
- Despite fewer fires overall, **fatalities increased**: from an annual average of ~22 pre-pandemic to ~28–35 in recent years (~35 in 2023) .

Regional & Urban Insights

Greater London saw **1,058 vehicle fires (Jan–Oct 2023)**; of these, **219 were EV-related** reddit.com+2honestjohn.co.uk+2reddit.com+2.

311 EV battery fires across UK in 2022–23, rising strongly into 2024–25 reddit.com.

⚡ Electric Vehicle & Lithium-Ion Battery Fires

- EV/battery-related fires in UK:
    - **390 (2022–23)**; **232 car fires** and **362 e-bike fires** in 2024 insurancebusinessmag.com.
    - UK fire services dealt with **1,330 lithium-ion battery incidents in 2024**, nearly **3 cases/day nationwide** fireservice.co.uk+2insurancebusinessmag.com+2theguardian.com+2.
- **211 e-bike/e-scooter fires** in 2024—a sharp rise from previous years—with **8 fatalities**, mostly in London theguardian.com.

Regional Hotspots (2023–24)

Based on insurance claims and reported incidents:

- **North West**: 106 vehicle fire claims
- **West Midlands**: 100
- **Greater London**: 100 committees.parliament.uk+15acorninsure.co.uk+15fireservice.co.uk+15bbc.co.uk

Summary

- **Annual incidents**: ~100,000 vehicle fires (19–20k serious road vehicle fires)
- **Deliberate**: ~60–65%; **accidental**: ~35–40%
- **Incidents trending down**, but **fatalities rising**
- **EV/battery fires increasing**, though still a small portion of overall figures
- **London and North West** among the most affected regions

Fire Detection and Suppression Systems in Vehicles

Fires in vehicles can escalate rapidly, making early detection and effective suppression critical to saving lives, reducing damage, and ensuring safe evacuation. In both private and commercial vehicles, fire detection and suppression systems provide a vital layer of safety—especially in high-risk sectors such as public transport, logistics, and emergency services.

1. Fire Detection Systems in Vehicles

Fire detection systems are designed to identify the early signs of fire—such as rising temperatures, smoke, or gas emissions—and alert occupants before the situation becomes critical.

Types of Vehicle Fire Detection Systems:

- **Heat Detectors**: Sense a rapid rise in temperature or temperatures above a preset threshold.

- **Smoke Detectors**: Detect particulate matter generated by combustion; commonly used in enclosed compartments like buses and RVs.
- **Flame Detectors**: Detect ultraviolet (UV) or infrared (IR) radiation from flames—often used in engine bays.
- **Gas Detectors**: Monitor for flammable or toxic gases (e.g., fuel vapour, hydrogen, CO) in electric or hybrid vehicles.
- **Thermal Cameras**: Used in advanced systems to monitor surface temperatures and detect overheating components before combustion.

Notification Methods:

- **Visual alerts** (dashboard warning lights)
- **Audible alarms** (buzzers or pre-recorded voice alerts)
- **Telematics notifications** (alerts sent to fleet control centres or emergency responders)

2. Fire Suppression Systems in Vehicles

Fire suppression systems work automatically or manually to extinguish fires in their early stages. These are especially important in commercial fleets, public transport, refrigerated trailers, and high-value or hazardous goods transport.

Types of Suppression Agents:

- **Dry Chemical Powders** (e.g., ABC powder): Fast-acting and effective on Class A (solids), B (flammable liquids), and C (electrical) fires.

- **Aqueous Film-Forming Foam (AFFF)**: Smothers and cools fuel fires, ideal for Class B (flammable liquid) fires.
- **Clean Agents** (e.g., FM-200, Novec 1230): Electrically non-conductive and leave no residue—ideal for sensitive equipment or EV battery compartments.
- **Water Mist Systems**: Use fine water droplets to cool surfaces and suppress fire without causing electrical shorts.

Suppression System Types:

- **Automatic Systems**:
    - Triggered by heat, smoke, or flame detection.
    - Common in engine compartments and enclosed cargo areas.
- **Manual Systems**:
    - Activated by the driver via a dashboard control or external pull handle.
- **Hybrid Systems**:
    - Combine automatic detection with manual override options for flexibility.

Maintenance and Inspection

Regular inspection and maintenance are essential for ensuring detection and suppression systems remain effective:

- **Monthly checks** of pressure gauges and indicator lights
- **Annual servicing** by qualified technicians
- **System testing** as per manufacturer's instructions or fleet safety policies

- **Documentation** of inspections, testing, and servicing for legal and insurance compliance

Legal and Regulatory Considerations (UK)

While not mandatory in all private vehicles, fire detection and suppression systems are:

- **Required or strongly recommended** in commercial vehicles, especially:
    - Passenger transport (e.g., buses and coaches)
    - Fuel and hazardous material carriers
    - Specialist vehicles (e.g., ambulances, mobile labs)
- **Recommended by bodies such as**:
    - The UK Department for Transport (DfT)
    - The British Standards Institution (BSI)
    - Insurance companies and fleet operators for risk mitigation
- **BS EN 28600** and **UNECE Regulation 107** provide guidance for systems used in buses and coaches.

Key Takeaways

- Fire detection systems provide early warning—critical for evacuation and safety.
- Suppression systems help extinguish fires before they spread.
- Commercial and high-risk vehicles benefit most from integrated fire safety systems.

- Regular maintenance is essential to ensure reliability.
- Employers and fleet operators may be legally required to install and maintain such systems in line with UK fire safety laws.

How to Use Fire Extinguishers in Vehicles

Vehicle fire extinguishers can help prevent a small fire from becoming a life-threatening emergency—but only if used **correctly**, **safely**, and **appropriately**.

🚨 **Before You Attempt to Use an Extinguisher:**

- Make sure **everyone is safely evacuated** from the vehicle.
- Only tackle **small, contained fires** (e.g. dashboard, upholstery, tyre or engine bay fires *without visible flames*).
- Never fight a fire if:
    - It's spreading rapidly
    - Involves fuel tanks or batteries
    - You are unsure or untrained

Know Your Fire Extinguisher

Type of Fire Extinguisher	Best For	Label Colour
Dry Powder (ABC)	Electrical, fuel, tyres, plastics	Blue
CO_2	Electrical components	Black
Foam (AFFF)	Flammable liquids like petrol/diesel	Cream

Type of Fire Extinguisher	Best For	Label Colour
Water	Solid combustibles (not electrics/fuel)	Red

For most vehicle fires, a **dry powder extinguisher (1–2kg)** is recommended

PASS Technique for Using a Fire Extinguisher

P – **Pull** the safety pin
A – **Aim** the nozzle at the base of the fire
S – **Squeeze** the handle to release the agent
S – **Sweep** side-to-side at the base of the flames until fire is extinguished ("Fundamentals: Safety/Infection Control Part 3 - Quizlet")

↻ Continue sweeping until the fire is fully out or the extinguisher is empty. Be ready to retreat if the fire re-ignites or intensifies.

Safe Usage Tips

- Stay **at least 1–2 metres** from the fire when discharging the extinguisher.
- Always keep a **clear escape route** behind you.
- Do **not** open the bonnet fully if the fire is in the engine bay—this feeds oxygen and may flare up. Instead, lift slightly and aim the nozzle through the gap.
- Avoid inhaling fumes—vehicle fires release **toxic gases**.

- Use extinguishers **only if trained** and when it's safe to do so.

After Use

- Move to a **safe distance**—reignition is possible.
- Report the fire to the **emergency services** even if extinguished.
- Arrange for the **extinguisher to be recharged or replaced**.
- Report the incident as per your workplace/fleet policy.

Legal and Practical Considerations (UK)

- Carrying a fire extinguisher is **not mandatory** in private vehicles but **strongly recommended**.
- **HGVs, minibuses, and commercial vehicles** are often required by law or insurance to carry a fire extinguisher (usually **2–6kg dry powder**, depending on size and risk).
- Extinguishers must be:
    - **Easily accessible** and securely mounted
    - **Checked monthly**
    - **Serviced annually** by a competent person

Quick Checklist

- Know the location and type of your extinguisher
- Check pressure and expiry date regularly
- Use only on small, early-stage fires
- Follow the PASS technique
- Always prioritise **evacuation and safety** over firefighting

Safe Handling of Flammable Liquids and Materials in Vehicles

Flammable substances—such as petrol, diesel, oil, gas cylinders, cleaning agents, paints, and aerosols—pose a serious fire risk when stored or transported in vehicles. Poor handling, improper storage, or accidental leaks can lead to ignition, explosions, and toxic exposure.

This guide outlines best practices for the safe transport, storage, and handling of flammable materials in vehicles, in line with UK fire safety regulations and HSE guidance.

1. Understand What Qualifies as Flammable

Common flammable materials in vehicles may include:

- **Fuels** (petrol, diesel, gas oil)
- **Compressed gases** (LPG, acetylene, butane)
- **Solvents and chemicals** (paint thinners, brake fluid)
- **Cleaning products** (alcohol-based sprays, degreasers)
- **Aerosols** (air fresheners, lubricants)
- **Combustible solids** (paper, cloths soaked in oil)

⚠ Check product Safety Data Sheets (SDS) for fire risk classification and handling instructions.

2. General Safety Rules for Handling

- Keep **flammable substances away from ignition sources** (e.g. smoking, sparks, heat, electrics).

- Ensure **adequate ventilation** when transporting or using flammable products.
- Wear **appropriate PPE** (e.g. gloves, eye protection, anti-static clothing).
- Do not decant flammable liquids **inside the vehicle** or in confined spaces.
- Avoid transporting flammable materials in the **passenger compartment**.

Safe Storage in the Vehicle

- Use **approved, sealed containers** for flammable liquids (e.g. UN-marked fuel cans).
- Store containers **upright and secured** to prevent tipping or leaks.
- Keep flammable items in a **dedicated storage compartment** or flame-retardant box if possible.
- Label containers clearly and visibly.
- Avoid overloading the vehicle and ensure **weight distribution** is safe.
- Do not store **excessive quantities**—only carry what is needed for operational purposes.

FIRE PREVENTION MEASURES

- Fit a **fire extinguisher** suitable for flammable liquid fires (e.g., **dry powder or foam**).
- Regularly inspect containers, hoses, and seals for **leaks or corrosion**.

- Install **spill kits** and absorbent materials to deal with small leaks.
- Use **non-sparking tools** if repairs or access to flammable substances are needed.
- Avoid **hot work** (e.g., welding, grinding) near stored flammable materials.

📓 5. Legal Requirements and Best Practice (UK)

- **COSHH Regulations**: Require safe handling of hazardous substances (including flammables).
- **ADR Regulations**: Apply if transporting flammable materials in quantities above threshold limits (e.g. by commercial operators).
- **Workplace Fire Safety Law**: Employers must assess risks and implement control measures for vehicle-based fire hazards.

Ensure compliance with the **Regulatory Reform (Fire Safety) Order 2005** and **Carriage of Dangerous Goods and Use of Transportable Pressure Equipment Regulations 2009** where applicable.

WHAT TO AVOID

- Leaving flammable materials in **hot vehicles** (e.g., parked in sun)
- Storing loose fuel containers or gas cylinders **unsecured**
- Mixing incompatible substances (e.g. fuel and oxidisers)
- Ignoring **warning signs** of leaks, fumes, or overheating
- Smoking or using open flames near stored flammables

7. Emergency Preparedness

- Know how to:
    - Identify and isolate a leak
    - Use a spill kit or absorbent
    - Evacuate and raise the alarm in case of fire
    - Inform emergency responders of the substances involved
- Keep emergency contact information and a brief **inventory of hazardous substances** in the vehicle.

Summary Checklist

Safety Measure	Completed? ✓
Only transport essential flammables	
Use proper containers and secure storage	
Avoid sources of heat or ignition	
Carry a suitable fire extinguisher	
Wear PPE when handling	
Follow legal limits and signage requirements	
Train all drivers in spill/fire procedures	

Fire Safety Responsibilities of Employed Drivers

Daily Safety Checks

Check for:

- Fuel, oil, or coolant leaks
- Exposed or damaged wiring
- Excessive engine or brake heat
- Obstructed or blocked exhausts

Use the Vehicle as Intended

Do not:

- Overload electrical sockets (e.g., with phone chargers)
- Carry unauthorised hazardous materials
- Leave the engine running when unattended in risk-prone areas

Carry Fire Safety Equipment (When Applicable)

Ensure availability and awareness of:

- **In-vehicle fire extinguisher** (if employer requires it)
- Knowledge of **fire extinguisher use** (e.g., PASS method)
- Emergency evacuation procedures

Report Defects Promptly

Notify the employer or fleet manager immediately if:

- Smoke, strange smells, or electrical faults are noticed
- The vehicle shows signs of overheating
- A near-miss, or minor fire-related issue occurs

Follow Employer Policies

Adhere to all fire safety-related procedures as outlined in:

- Driver handbooks
- Safety inductions
- Fleet operating policies

Summary of Legal Responsibilities

Duty	Description	Relevant Law
Daily vehicle checks	Spot fire risks early	HSWA 1974, PUWER
Safe operation	Use equipment properly, avoid hazards	PUWER, Road Traffic Act 1988
Report risks	Inform management of defects/faults	MHSWR 1999
Follow training & policy	Adhere to employer's safety systems	HSWA 1974
Use equipment responsibly	Fire extinguishers, emergency kit, electronics	PUWER

Consequences of Non-Compliance

- **Fines or Prosecution** (for the driver or employer)
- **Increased risk of injury or death**
- **Invalid insurance claims**
- **Corporate liability under manslaughter laws**
- **Loss of employment or driving license**

Remember: Under UK law, employed drivers are not just operators—they are active participants in maintaining vehicle safety. Fire prevention begins with daily awareness and responsible action.

\Vehicle Fire Safety Checklist (Daily Use)

Item	Check	Notes
Electrical wiring and battery terminals	☐	Look for fraying, corrosion, or exposed wires
Fuel lines, tank, and seals	☐	Check for leaks or fuel odour
Fire extinguisher present and inspected	☐	Must be in date, correctly mounted, and accessible
Fire exits and escape doors (if applicable)	☐	Ensure they are unlocked and unblocked
Flammable items stored safely	☐	No loose petrol cans, aerosols, or flammable cargo
Extinguisher usage training up to date	☐	At least annually or per company policy
Engine temperature and warning lights	☐	Address any irregularities before departure

Item	Check	Notes
Charging equipment (EVs) undamaged	☐	Check cables, sockets, and connections

Post-Incident Checklist for Drivers

Task	Completed?
Ensured all passengers were evacuated safely	☐
Called emergency services and provided accurate location	☐
Used fire extinguisher safely if appropriate	☐
Reported the incident to employer or fleet manager	☐
Completed a written incident report	☐
Supported the post-incident investigation if required	☐

Tip: Regular Fire Safety Drills

- Conduct vehicle fire response **drills** at least every 6–12 months.
- Use scenario-based training with mock extinguishers or VR tools.
- Include **emergency contact procedures**, evacuation drills, and extinguisher simulations.

Final Message for Drivers:

Every second counts in a vehicle fire.
Your **preparedness, knowledge**, and **calm response** can mean the difference between safety and disaster. Don't wait for a real emergency—train, check, and stay alert.

Vehicle Fires in the UK: Intentional Fires – Arson, Fraud, and Criminal Cover-up

Intentional vehicle fires represent a significant proportion of all fire-related incidents in the UK. These are not accidents, but **deliberate acts** often connected to **criminal activity, financial gain, or malicious intent**.

UK Statistics on Intentional Vehicle Fires

According to the UK Home Office and Fire and Rescue Services data:

- **Approximately 65%** of all vehicle fires in the UK are suspected to be **deliberately started**.
- That translates to over **65,000 intentional vehicle fires** annually—almost **180 every day**.
- Many occur in **urban areas**, particularly in regions with higher crime rates, youth unemployment, and social deprivation.
- These incidents are often linked to:
    - **Theft and disposal of stolen vehicles**
    - **Insurance fraud schemes**
    - **Retaliation, gang-related activity, or vandalism**

- o **Evidence destruction** (e.g. following burglaries or violent crimes)

Common Motives for Intentional Vehicle Fires

1. Arson for Vandalism or Retaliation

- Typically involves **youths or gangs** targeting vehicles for anti-social reasons.
- Common in areas with **limited CCTV surveillance or poor lighting**.
- May be used to **intimidate** individuals or communities.

2. Insurance Fraud (Vehicle Arson Fraud)

- Owners may intentionally destroy a vehicle to:
    - o Avoid costly repairs or finance repayments.
    - o Claim a **payout for a 'total loss'**.
- Fraudsters may:
    - o Stage the fire to resemble an accident.
    - o Abandon the vehicle in remote areas.
- This is a **criminal offence**, punishable by prosecution and imprisonment.

3. Criminal Cover-Up

- Vehicles may be torched to **eliminate forensic evidence** following crimes such as:
    - o **Armed robbery**
    - o **Drug transportation**
    - o **Assault or abduction**

- Fire destroys fingerprints, DNA, CCTV systems, and other physical clues.

Legal Consequences in the UK

Intentional vehicle fires fall under serious offences, including:

Offence	Legal Classification	Penalty
Arson	Indictable offence	Life imprisonment (if endangering life)
Insurance fraud	Criminal fraud	Up to 10 years in prison
Conspiracy to commit arson	Criminal conspiracy	Up to life imprisonment
Criminal damage	Either-way offence	Up to 10 years' imprisonment

Additionally, individuals convicted of insurance fraud or criminal arson may face:

- Civil penalties and compensation orders
- Driving disqualification
- Loss of employment or professional registration
- Public naming and reputational harm

Preventive Measures for Drivers and Operators

To reduce the risk of intentional fires:

- **Park in secure, well-lit areas** with CCTV surveillance.

- Use **steering locks, immobilisers, and vehicle tracking systems**.
- Avoid leaving **valuable items** or identifying documents inside vehicles.
- **Report suspicious behaviour** near vehicles, especially at depots, car parks, or roadside laybys.
- Ensure company or fleet vehicles are:
    - **Always locked when unattended**
    - **Monitored through GPS or telematics**
- Maintain up-to-date **insurance and inspection records** to help prevent fraudulent accusations.

What to Do If You Suspect Arson

If you suspect your vehicle or another has been targeted:

1. **Do not attempt to approach the fire**—keep a safe distance.
2. **Call 999** and report the fire immediately.
3. **Avoid touching or moving the vehicle** before police or fire services arrive.
4. **Preserve any CCTV footage or witness accounts**.
5. **Cooperate fully** with fire investigators and police to support criminal proceedings.

For Fleet Managers and Employers

- Implement **incident reporting protocols** for suspected arson.
- Train staff on **vehicle fire prevention and emergency response**.

- Liaise with local police and fire services to conduct **risk assessments** in vulnerable areas.
- Review insurance policies for fraud protection and arson cover.

Remember:

Intentional vehicle fires are not just property crimes—they endanger lives, disrupt public services, and place immense strain on emergency resources.

Reporting suspicious activity, securing vehicles, and understanding the risks can save lives and protect livelihoods.

Responsibilities of Employers under UK Fire Safety Law

Under current UK fire safety legislation, particularly the **Regulatory Reform (Fire Safety) Order 2005**, employers (referred to as the "Responsible Person") have a **legal duty** to ensure the safety of employees, visitors, and anyone who may be affected by fire risks in the workplace. These responsibilities include, but are not limited to:

1. Fire Risk Assessment (FRA)

- Employers must carry out a **suitable and sufficient fire risk assessment** of the workplace.
- The assessment must identify potential fire hazards, assess who may be at risk, evaluate current fire safety measures, and determine what improvements are necessary.
- Risk assessments must be **reviewed regularly**—especially if there are significant changes to the premises, operations, or workforce.
- Employers may appoint a **competent person** to assist, but **legal responsibility remains with the employer**.

2. Provision of Information

- Employers must provide clear and accessible information on **identified fire risks** and **preventive measures** to all staff, including:
    - Fire evacuation procedures
    - Location and use of fire extinguishers

- Alarm systems and escape routes
- Information must also be shared with **temporary staff, contractors, and visitors** as appropriate.
- **Fire safety signage** (e.g., emergency exit signs, fire extinguisher locations) must be in place, clearly visible, and compliant with UK safety standards.

3. Fire Safety Training

- Employees must receive **adequate and regular fire safety training**, including:
    - What to do in the event of a fire
    - How to raise the alarm
    - Use of fire extinguishers (if appropriate)
    - Fire marshal or warden responsibilities (for designated individuals)
- Training must be provided:
    - **On induction**
    - **At regular intervals** thereafter
    - **Whenever significant changes** occur (e.g., to the building layout, personnel, or fire procedures)
- Training must be **recorded and documented**.

4. Consultation with Employees

- Employers are required to **consult with employees or their safety representatives** on fire safety matters, including:
    - Risk assessment findings
    - Fire evacuation strategies
    - Fire safety policies and updates

- Involving employees helps improve awareness, compliance, and fire prevention culture across the organisation.

5. Maintenance of Fire Safety Systems and Equipment

- Employers must ensure all fire safety systems and equipment are **maintained in good working order**, including:
    - Fire alarms and detectors
    - Emergency lighting
    - Fire doors
    - Fire extinguishers
- Maintenance should follow the manufacturer's guidance and be performed by **competent persons**.
- Records of **testing, inspections, servicing, and repairs** must be kept.

6. Record-Keeping and Compliance

- Employers in **non-domestic premises** with **five or more employees** must:
    - Keep written records of fire risk assessments
    - Record training and maintenance logs
    - Document roles, responsibilities, and policies relating to fire safety
- These records may be **inspected by the local Fire and Rescue Authority** during routine audits or following an incident.

Legal Consequences of Non-Compliance

Failure to comply with UK fire safety legislation can result in:

- **Enforcement notices**
- **Prohibition notices**
- **Prosecution**
- **Unlimited fines**
- In serious cases, **imprisonment** for the responsible person

Post-Fire Protocols: Incident Reporting and Investigation

For Vehicle Fires – With Emphasis on UK Requirements

Once a vehicle fire has been extinguished or contained, it is crucial to follow structured **post-incident procedures** to ensure safety, regulatory compliance, and future prevention. In the UK, vehicle operators—especially those in commercial or public service sectors—must follow specific reporting, documentation, and investigation protocols.

1. Immediate Actions Following a Fire

After ensuring everyone is safe and emergency services have been contacted:

- **Do not re-enter the vehicle** until cleared as safe.
- Move a safe distance away from the vehicle—**reignition is possible**.
- **Preserve the scene** for investigation (do not tamper with equipment or evidence).

- Notify:
    - Line manager or transport supervisor
    - Fire and Rescue Service (if not already informed)
    - Police, if the fire is suspected to be deliberate or caused injury

2. Incident Reporting Requirements (UK)

All vehicle fire incidents must be reported in line with workplace and regulatory expectations:

For Commercial and Work Vehicles:

- Complete your organisation's **internal incident report** (ideally within 24 hours).
- Notify your **fleet or transport manager** and **Health & Safety officer**.
- Record key details:
    - Date, time, location
    - Vehicle registration and type
    - Description of incident and sequence of events
    - Suspected cause (if known)
    - Actions taken (extinguisher used, emergency services called, evacuation)
    - Any injuries, damage, or environmental impact
- If the vehicle is part of a commercial or public fleet, include **maintenance logs and inspection history** as part of the report.

📝 Statutory Reporting May Be Required If:

- The fire resulted in **injury, fatality, or hospitalisation**.
- Dangerous goods were involved.
- There was **significant damage** or environmental contamination.
- It qualifies as a **RIDDOR-reportable incident** (see Section 3).

3. Legal and Regulatory Reporting Obligations (UK)

RIDDOR (Reporting of Injuries, Diseases and Dangerous Occurrences Regulations 2013)

You must report to the HSE (Health and Safety Executive) if the fire:

- Results in a **work-related injury requiring >7 days off**
- Leads to **hospital admission**
- Involves **explosions or incidents with flammable substances** in a work setting

Who Reports?
The **employer, responsible person**, or **fleet operator** must report via HSE's RIDDOR Portal.

4. Internal Investigation

An internal investigation must be conducted to determine:

- The **root cause** of the fire (e.g., mechanical fault, human error, arson)
- Whether the correct **response procedures** were followed

- Any **failures in equipment, maintenance, or training**
- **Corrective actions** to prevent recurrence

Steps to Follow:

1. **Gather evidence**: photographs, dashcam footage, driver statements, extinguisher use
2. **Interview witnesses** and involved staff
3. **Review maintenance records**, inspection logs, and fire extinguisher servicing
4. **Consult with fire safety or vehicle engineers**, if required

5. Documentation and Record-Keeping

Maintain detailed records for:

- Incident reports
- RIDDOR submissions (if applicable)
- Investigation outcomes
- Equipment and vehicle inspection reports
- Fire extinguisher usage/replacement logs
- Training records (relevant to fire safety and emergency response)

Records must be kept for **a minimum of 3 years** in line with HSE and insurance requirements. Longer retention may be required for fleet operators or high-risk industries.

6. Review and Continuous Improvement

- Conduct a **lessons-learned session** with relevant personnel.

- Update:
  - **Risk assessments** (especially if a mechanical or systemic fault is found)
  - **Training protocols**
  - **Emergency procedures**
- Consider retraining if response protocols were **not followed correctly**.

7. Insurance Notification

- Notify your **insurance provider immediately** after the incident.
- Provide:
  - Fire and police reference numbers
  - Investigation summary
  - Repair estimates and supporting documents
- Failure to report promptly may affect **insurance claims or liability assessments**.

Post-Fire Protocol Checklist

Task	Responsible Party	Completed?
Secure the scene	Driver / Supervisor	☐
Notify emergency services	Driver / Witness	☐
Submit internal incident report	Driver / Manager	☐
Notify insurance provider	Fleet Manager	☐

Task	Responsible Party	Completed?
Report to HSE (if RIDDOR applies)	Safety Officer	☐
Conduct internal investigation	Appointed Investigator	☐
Record all findings and actions	H&S Officer	☐
Update risk assessments	Management	☐

Responsibilities of Employees under UK Fire Safety Law

Under the **Regulatory Reform (Fire Safety) Order 2005**, all employees have a **legal duty** to take reasonable care for their safety and the safety of others who may be affected by fire risks in the workplace. Fire safety is a shared responsibility, and cooperation between employees and employers is essential to maintain a safe environment.

The key responsibilities of employees include:

1. Awareness of Fire Safety Procedures and Systems

- Employees must familiarise themselves with the location and operation of:
    - Fire alarms and call points
    - Escape routes and emergency exits
    - Assembly points
    - Firefighting equipment (e.g., extinguishers—if trained and appropriate to use)
- Employees should **immediately report** any obstructions, faults, or concerns related to fire exits, alarms, or equipment.

2. Adherence to Fire Safety Policies

- Employees must **read, understand, and follow** the fire safety policies and procedures provided by the employer.
- These policies may include:
    - Site-specific fire evacuation plans

- Personal emergency evacuation plans (PEEPs) where applicable
- Fire prevention measures (e.g., safe storage of flammable substances, no smoking areas)

3. Participation in Fire Drills

- Employees are expected to **participate fully and responsibly in scheduled fire drills**.
- Fire drills are required by law and provide practice in:
  - Evacuating promptly
  - Assembling at the designated point
  - Understanding the roles of fire marshals or wardens
- Employees should treat drills **as real events** and raise concerns if issues arise during the drill.

4. Attendance at Fire Safety Training

- Employees must **attend fire safety training** sessions as required by their role or the nature of the workplace.
- Training ensures staff are confident in:
  - Identifying fire hazards
  - Responding to alarms
  - Knowing what actions to take in a fire emergency
- Training must be repeated periodically and after any significant changes to the workplace, processes, or legislation.

5. Cooperating with the Employer and Safety Representatives

- Employees have a duty to:

- Cooperate with the employer's fire safety arrangements
- Follow lawful instructions relating to fire safety
- Support investigations into fire-related incidents or near misses
- Engage in consultations or feedback processes when reviewing fire safety procedures

6. Reporting Hazards or Deficiencies

- Employees must **promptly report any fire safety concerns**, including:
    - Faulty alarms or extinguishers
    - Blocked escape routes
    - Improper storage of flammable materials
    - Unfamiliar persons or suspicious activity in fire-sensitive areas
- Reports should be made to the designated fire safety officer, line manager, or via the organisation's incident reporting system.

7. Awareness from Day One

- Fire safety information must be provided to all employees **on their first day of employment** as part of the induction process.
- Employees should also be kept informed of:
    - Any updates or reviews to fire safety policies and procedures

- Changes to the building, operations, or staffing that may affect evacuation plans

Legal Context

Failure by employees to follow fire safety protocols may result in:

- Disciplinary action by the employer
- Legal liability in cases of negligence
- Increased risk to life, health, and property

Causes of Fire in the Workplace

Workplace fires can cause significant injury, loss of life, property damage, and disruption of business operations. Compliance with fire safety legislation—including the **Regulatory Reform (Fire Safety) Order 2005**—is essential for employers and responsible persons. The most common causes of fire in the workplace include:

1. Deliberate Acts (Arson)

- Arson remains a leading cause of workplace fires. This may involve deliberate ignition by disgruntled employees, ex-employees, or intruders.
- Inadequate security measures or poor access control can increase vulnerability.

Prevention Measures:

- Install security lighting and CCTV.
- Secure external waste bins away from the building.
- Encourage staff to report suspicious activity.

2. Electrical Faults and Misuse

Electrical fires are a major risk in commercial environments due to the widespread use of equipment and appliances.

Common faults and risks include:

- Overloaded extension leads and multi-plug adaptors.
- Damaged or exposed wiring.

- Loose connections or faulty sockets and outlets.
- Poorly maintained or outdated appliances.
- Portable heaters placed near flammable items.

Control Measures:

- Conduct regular **Portable Appliance Testing (PAT)**.
- Use circuit breakers and Residual Current Devices (RCDs).
- Avoid daisy-chaining extension leads.
- Engage a competent electrician for installations and repairs.

3. Smoking-Related Incidents

- Fires can be caused by careless disposal of smoking materials in unauthorised areas or inadequate smoking facilities.

Control Measures:

- Designate and clearly signpost smoking areas.
- Provide proper fire-resistant disposal bins (e.g., sand buckets or sealed receptacles).
- Implement and enforce a workplace **No Smoking Policy** in compliance with the **Smoke-free (Premises and Enforcement) Regulations 2006**.

4. Heating Equipment

- Misuse of portable or fixed heating equipment is a frequent ignition source.

Common risks include:

- Heaters placed too close to combustible materials.
- Covered vents or airflow obstructions.
- Inadequate maintenance.

Preventative Steps:

- Ensure heaters have automatic shut-off features.
- Maintain clear space around heaters (at least 1 metre).
- Perform regular inspections.

5. Hot Work (Welding, Cutting, Grinding)

- Activities involving open flames or sparks can ignite surrounding materials if not properly managed.

Control Measures:

- Conduct a **Hot Work Risk Assessment** before starting work.
- Use fire-retardant blankets or screens.
- Issue a **Hot Work Permit** with a designated fire watch period after work completion.
- Keep fire extinguishers and fire blankets nearby.

6. Improper Storage of Flammable and Combustible Materials

Many workplaces use or store flammable liquids and combustible solids that, when mishandled, greatly increase fire risk.

Flammable Liquids:

Examples:

- Alcohols (e.g., isopropanol, ethanol)
- Petrol
- Solvents and adhesives

Precautions:

- Store in approved, ventilated containers.
- Keep away from ignition sources and heat.
- Follow **COSHH Regulations** for handling hazardous substances.

Combustible Materials:

Examples:

- Paper and cardboard
- Wood
- Plastics and rubber

Precautions:

- Store in designated, clutter-free areas.
- Do not block emergency exits or fire escape routes.
- Dispose of waste regularly and responsibly.

Electrical Fires: Key Hazards

Electrical fires are frequently caused by the following:

- **Faulty Sockets and Outlets:** Overheating from poor contacts or age.
- **Damaged Light Fittings:** Loose wires or exposed components.
- **Overused Extension Leads:** Overloading circuits beyond safe limits.
- **Portable Heaters:** Often improperly placed or used near flammables.
- **Outdated or Poorly Installed Wiring:** Cannot handle modern electrical loads.
- **Old or Faulty Appliances:** Worn components may spark or overheat.

Mitigation Tips:

- Install Residual Current Devices (RCDs).
- Label high-load circuits.
- Maintain up-to-date electrical inspection records (EICR every 5 years for most workplaces).

▪ Fire Safety Compliance Essentials (UK)

To comply with the **Regulatory Reform (Fire Safety) Order 2005**, all employers must:

- Conduct a **Fire Risk Assessment** and review it regularly.
- Provide **suitable fire detection and alarm systems**.

- Install and maintain **fire-fighting equipment** (e.g., extinguishers).
- Ensure all **escape routes and exits are unobstructed** and well-signposted.
- Appoint and train **Fire Marshals or Wardens**.
- Conduct regular **fire drills and staff training**.
- Display clear **fire action notices** and evacuation maps.

Causes of Fire in the Workplace

Workplace fires can cause significant injury, loss of life, property damage, and disruption of business operations. Compliance with fire safety legislation—including the **Regulatory Reform (Fire Safety) Order 2005**—is essential for employers and responsible persons. The most common causes of fire in the workplace include:

1. Deliberate Acts (Arson)

- Arson remains a leading cause of workplace fires. This may involve deliberate ignition by disgruntled employees, ex-employees, or intruders.
- Inadequate security measures or poor access control can increase vulnerability.

Prevention Measures:

- Install security lighting and CCTV.
- Secure external waste bins away from the building.
- Encourage staff to report suspicious activity.

2. Electrical Faults and Misuse

- Electrical fires are a major risk in commercial environments due to the widespread use of equipment and appliances.

Common faults and risks include:

- Overloaded extension leads and multi-plug adaptors.
- Damaged or exposed wiring.
- Loose connections or faulty sockets and outlets.
- Poorly maintained or outdated appliances.
- Portable heaters placed near flammable items.

Control Measures:

- Conduct regular **Portable Appliance Testing (PAT)**.
- Use circuit breakers and Residual Current Devices (RCDs).
- Avoid daisy-chaining extension leads.
- Engage a competent electrician for installations and repairs.

3. Smoking-Related Incidents

- Fires can be caused by careless disposal of smoking materials in unauthorised areas or inadequate smoking facilities.

Control Measures:

- Designate and clearly signpost smoking areas.
- Provide proper fire-resistant disposal bins (e.g., sand buckets or sealed receptacles).

- Implement and enforce a workplace **No Smoking Policy** in compliance with the **Smoke-free (Premises and Enforcement) Regulations 2006**.

4. Heating Equipment

- Misuse of portable or fixed heating equipment is a frequent ignition source.

Common risks include:

- Heaters placed too close to combustible materials.
- Covered vents or airflow obstructions.
- Inadequate maintenance.

Preventative Steps:

- Ensure heaters have automatic shut-off features.
- Maintain clear space around heaters (at least 1 metre).
- Perform regular inspections.

5. Hot Work (Welding, Cutting, Grinding)

- Activities involving open flames or sparks can ignite surrounding materials if not properly managed.

Control Measures:

- Conduct a **Hot Work Risk Assessment** before starting work.
- Use fire-retardant blankets or screens.

- Issue a **Hot Work Permit** with a designated fire watch period after work completion.
- Keep fire extinguishers and fire blankets nearby.

6. Improper Storage of Flammable and Combustible Materials

- Many workplaces use or store flammable liquids and combustible solids that, when mishandled, greatly increase fire risk.

Flammable Liquids:

Examples:

- Alcohols (e.g., isopropanol, ethanol)
- Petrol
- Solvents and adhesives

Precautions:

- Store in approved, ventilated containers.
- Keep away from ignition sources and heat.
- Follow **COSHH Regulations** for handling hazardous substances.

Combustible Materials:

Examples:

- Paper and cardboard
- Wood
- Plastics and rubber

Precautions:

- Store in designated, clutter-free areas.
- Do not block emergency exits or fire escape routes.
- Dispose of waste regularly and responsibly.

Electrical Fires: Key Hazards

Electrical fires are frequently caused by the following:

- **Faulty Sockets and Outlets:** Overheating from poor contacts or age.
- **Damaged Light Fittings:** Loose wires or exposed components.
- **Overused Extension Leads:** Overloading circuits beyond safe limits.
- **Portable Heaters:** Often improperly placed or used near flammables.
- **Outdated or Poorly Installed Wiring:** Cannot handle modern electrical loads.
- **Old or Faulty Appliances:** Worn components may spark or overheat.

Mitigation Tips:

- Install Residual Current Devices (RCDs).
- Label high-load circuits.
- Maintain up-to-date electrical inspection records (EICR every 5 years for most workplaces).

Fire Safety Compliance Essentials (UK)

To comply with the **Regulatory Reform (Fire Safety) Order 2005**, all employers must:

- Conduct a **Fire Risk Assessment** and review it regularly.
- Provide **suitable fire detection and alarm systems**.
- Install and maintain **fire-fighting equipment** (e.g., extinguishers).
- Ensure all **escape routes and exits are unobstructed** and well-signposted.
- Appoint and train **Fire Marshals or Wardens**.
- Conduct regular **fire drills and staff training**.
- Display clear **fire action notices** and evacuation maps.

Would you like this content formatted for a training manual, slide deck, or printable handout?

Causes of Motor Vehicle Fires

Motor vehicle fires pose significant risks to life, property, and the environment. Whether occurring in commercial fleets, public roadways, or workplace transport operations, understanding and mitigating these causes is critical for compliance with UK safety legislation and for preventing injury and loss.

1. Mechanical Failures

Overheating, friction, and poor maintenance are frequent mechanical contributors to vehicle fires.

Key examples:

- Overheated engines due to failed cooling systems.
- Leaking gaskets causing oil to drip onto hot surfaces.
- Seized bearings or brake components generating high heat.

Control Measures:

- Conduct routine mechanical inspections.
- Ensure cooling systems (radiators, hoses, fans) are functioning correctly.
- Replace worn or damaged components promptly.
- Comply with manufacturer service schedules.

2. Electrical Faults

Electrical malfunctions are among the leading causes of vehicle fires, especially in modern vehicles with complex systems.

Common risks:

- Damaged or corroded wiring harnesses.
- Poorly installed aftermarket electronics (e.g., alarms, stereos).
- Short circuits from battery terminals or alternators.
- Overloaded power sockets or charging ports.

Control Measures:

- Regular electrical system checks by qualified personnel.
- Use only manufacturer-approved or CE-marked components.
- Ensure correct fuse ratings are used.
- Inspect and secure battery connections; avoid terminal corrosion.

3. Fuel System Leaks

Fuel (petrol or diesel) is highly flammable. Leaks in the fuel delivery system can lead to vapour buildup and ignition, especially near heat sources.

Risks include:

- Cracked fuel lines or loose fittings.
- Leaky fuel injectors or carburettors.
- Fuel spills during refuelling, especially near ignition sources.

Control Measures:

- Immediately repair or replace compromised components.
- Only refuel when the engine is off and cool.

- Ensure ventilation when working near fuel systems.

4. Contact with Hot Surfaces

Combustible materials may ignite if they come into contact with heated engine parts or exhaust components.

Common examples:

- Oil, grease, or leaves accumulating near exhaust manifolds.
- Insulation or bodywork sagging onto heat shields.
- Underbody vegetation from off-road use.

Control Measures:

- Regularly clean the engine bay and undercarriage.
- Ensure heat shields and covers are intact and secured.
- Avoid parking on dry grass or flammable surfaces after driving.

💥 5. Collisions and Impact Damage

Vehicle crashes can rupture fuel lines, damage batteries, or cause short circuits, leading to post-collision fires.

Risks include:

- Fuel tank ruptures.
- Crushed electrical components.
- Brake fluid or transmission fluid leaks ignited by friction.

Control Measures:

- Ensure vehicles are fitted with impact-absorbing structures where possible.
- Train staff in post-collision fire response and evacuation procedures.
- Equip fleet vehicles with suitable **fire extinguishers (BS EN3 approved)**.

🛠 6. Poor Maintenance or Tampering

Neglecting vehicle maintenance or unauthorised modifications can introduce significant fire risks.

Examples:

- Use of incorrect replacement parts.
- Missing heat shields or engine bay seals.
- Bypass of fuses or safety relays.

Control Measures:

- Follow manufacturer maintenance guidance.
- Avoid DIY modifications.
- Keep accurate servicing records, especially in commercial vehicle operations (as required under PUWER).

7. Hazardous Materials and Cargo

Vehicles transporting flammable or reactive substances are at higher risk, especially if the cargo is not secured correctly or labelled.

Examples:

- Transporting fuel, paint, gas cylinders, or chemicals.
- Incompatible chemicals reacting during transit.
- Leaking containers or damaged packaging.

Control Measures:

- Adhere to **ADR (Carriage of Dangerous Goods by Road) regulations**.
- Clearly label all hazardous materials.
- Train drivers in spill and fire response procedures.
- Secure cargo using fire-resistant barriers where required.

8. Human Error and Negligence

Deliberate or careless behaviour can also be a major contributor to vehicle fires.

Risks include:

- Smoking inside or near vehicles with flammable contents.
- Improper refuelling or use of fuel containers.
- Discarding matches or cigarettes near vents or fuel tanks.

Control Measures:

- Enforce no-smoking policies in and around vehicles.
- Provide driver training on fire prevention.
- Use signage to indicate fire risks in refuelling areas.

Classes of Fire (UK Classification – BS EN 2:1992)

Understanding fire classes is essential for selecting the appropriate fire extinguisher and ensuring a safe and effective response in an emergency. Each class represents the type of fuel involved.

Class A – Solid Combustible Materials

Description: Fires involving **solid, organic materials** that are not metals.

Examples:

- Wood
- Paper
- Textiles
- Plastics
- Cardboard
- Furniture

Extinguishing Methods:

- **Water** (cools the burning material)
- **Foam**
- **Dry Powder**
- **Wet Chemical (limited use)**

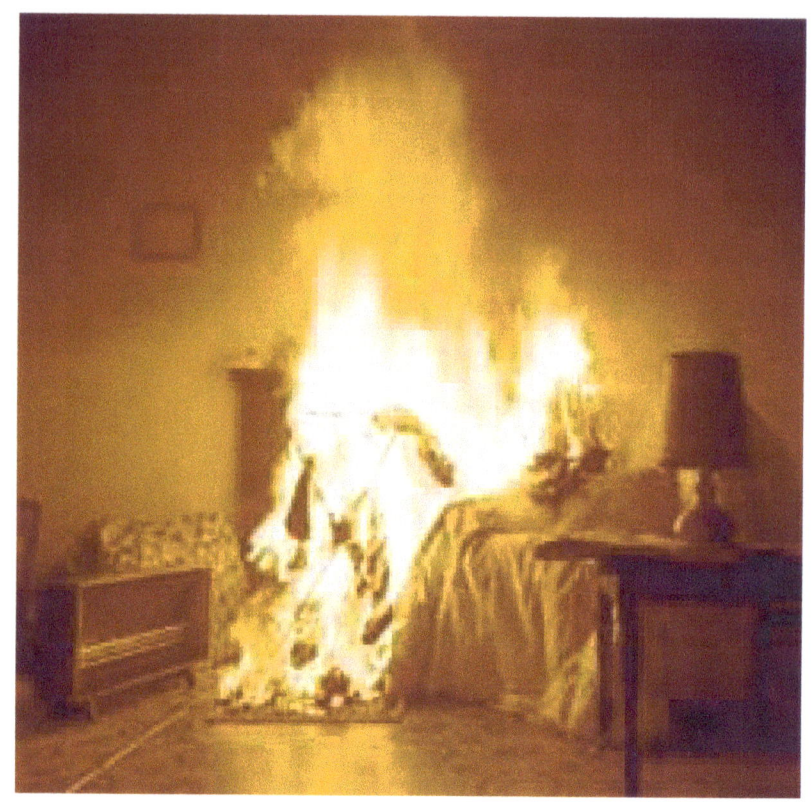

Class B – Flammable Liquids

Description: Fires involving **flammable or combustible liquids**.

Examples:

- Petrol
- Diesel
- Paint
- Alcohol
- Oils (except cooking oils – see Class F)

Extinguishing Methods:

- **Foam** (smothers the fire)
- **Dry Powder**
- CO_2
- **Never use water** (can spread the flammable liquid)

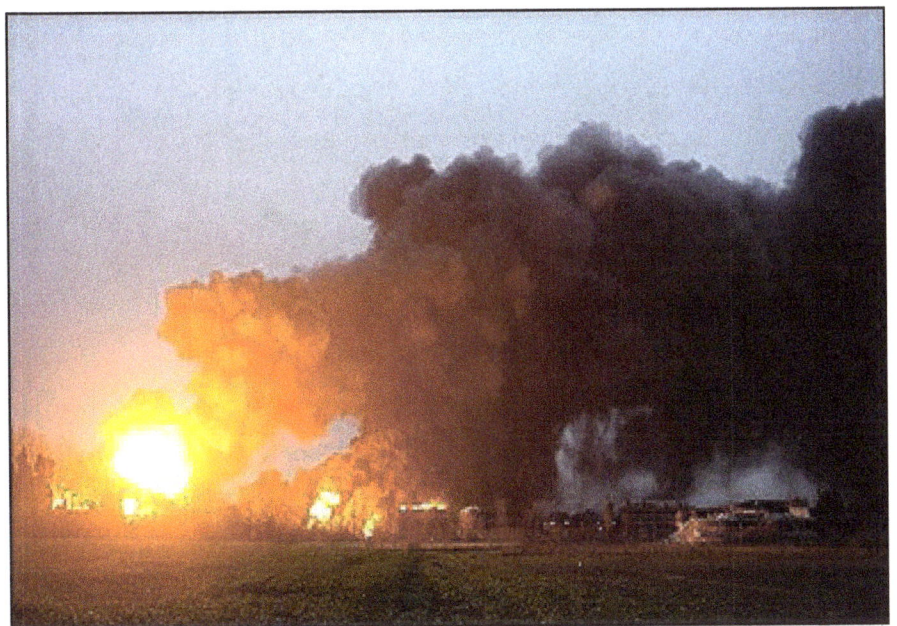

Class C – Flammable Gases

Description: Fires involving **flammable gases**.

Examples:

- Propane
- Butane
- Methane

- Acetylene

Extinguishing Methods:

- **Dry Powder**
- Stop the gas supply **before** extinguishing
- Specialist suppression systems may be needed

Important Note: Do **not** extinguish without isolating the gas supply — doing so may cause unburned gas to accumulate and lead to an explosion.

Class D – Combustible Metals

Description: Fires involving **flammable metals**.

Examples:

- Magnesium
- Titanium
- Aluminium shavings
- Lithium
- Potassium
- Sodium

Extinguishing Methods:

- **Specialist Dry Powder Extinguishers (e.g., L2 or M28)**
- **Do not use water or CO_2** — can cause violent reactions

Common Settings: Laboratories, manufacturing, metal workshops

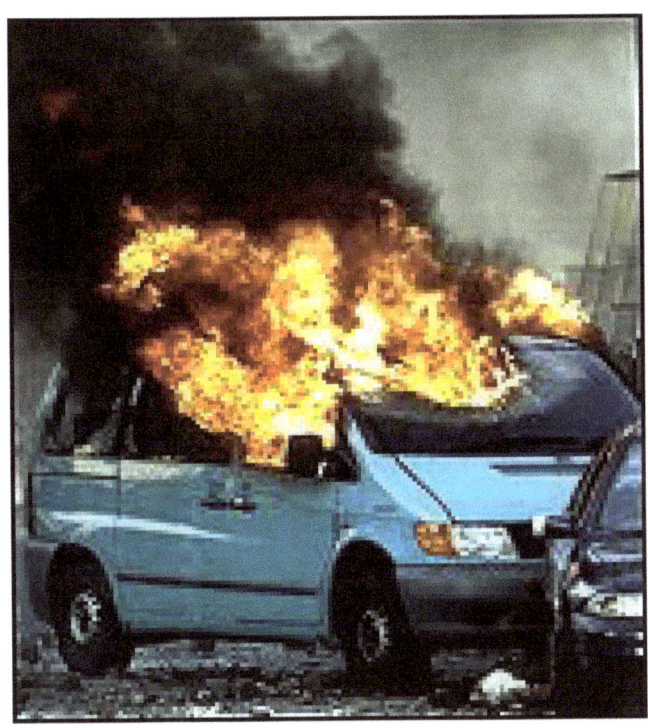

Electrical Fires (formerly Class E – Obsolete)

Description: Fires **involving or caused by electrical equipment**.

Examples:

- Overloaded circuits
- Faulty appliances
- Electric panels
- Servers or data equipment

UK Note: **Electrical fires are not classified as a separate class (Class E is obsolete)** but are instead identified as an **additional hazard**. Once the electrical source is isolated, the fire is classified by its fuel (e.g., Class A or B).

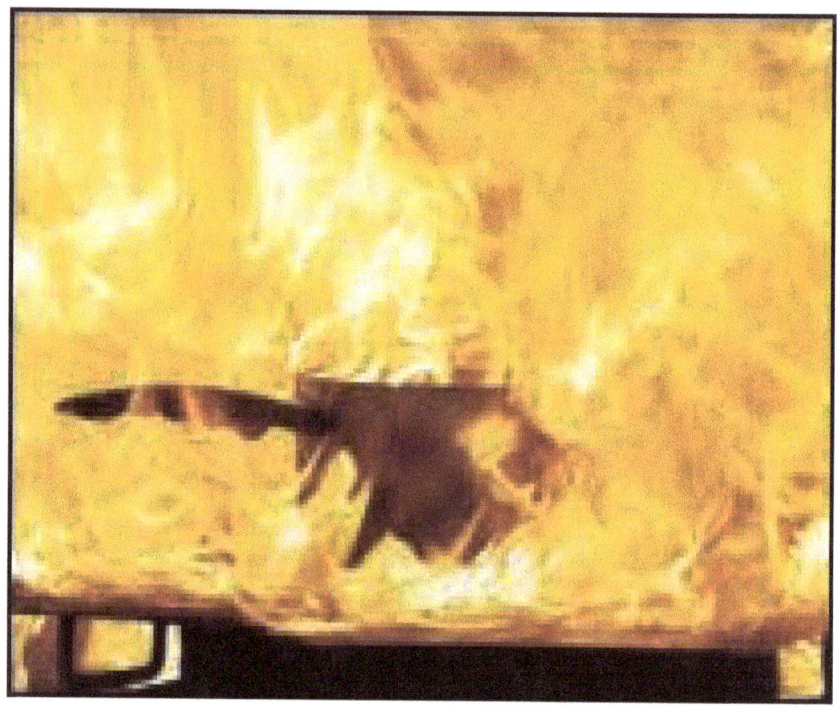

Extinguishing Methods:

- CO_2
- **Dry Powder**
- **Do not use water or foam** on live electricals
- **Always isolate the Power Supply First**, if safe to do so.

Class F – Cooking Oils and Fats

Description: Fires involving **high-temperature cooking oils or fats**, typically in deep-fat fryers.

Examples:

- Vegetable oil
- Lard
- Commercial cooking fat

Extinguishing Methods:

- **Wet Chemical Extinguishers** (cool and chemically suppress the flames)
- **Fire blankets** (small pan fires only)

Do not use:

- Water (will cause violent splashing and fire spread)
- Foam or standard dry powder (ineffective and dangerous)

Fire Extinguisher Types & Their Uses

Quick Reference Guide for Vehicle Drivers

Extinguisher Type	Class A <small>Ordinary Combustibles</small>	Class B <small>Flammable Liquids</small>	Class C <small>Flammable Gases</small>	Class D <small>Combustible Metals</small>	Electrical Fires	Class F <small>Cooking Oils & Fats</small>
Water	✓ Suitable	✗ Not suitable	✗ Not suitable	✗ Not suitable	✗ Not suitable	✗ Not suitable
Foam	✓ Suitable	✓ Suitable	✗ Not suitable	✗ Not suitable	✗ Not suitable	✗ Not suitable
Dry Powder	✓ Suitable	✓ Suitable	✓ Suitable	✓ *Specific types	✓ Suitable	✗ Not suitable
CO₂	✗ Not suitable	✓ Suitable	✓ Suitable	✗ Not suitable	✓ Suitable	✗ Not suitable
Wet Chemical	✓ Suitable	✗ Not suitable	✗ Not suitable	✗ Not suitable	✗ Not suitable	✓ Suitable

✓ Key:

- ✓ **Suitable** – Effective for this type of fire
- ✗ **Not Suitable** – Do not use for this type of fire
- ✓ *Specific types only* – Dry powder for Class D must be designed for specific metals (e.g. magnesium)

Notes for Drivers:

- Always check the **label and type** of extinguisher before use.
- Use the **PASS technique**: **Pull** the pin, **Aim** at the base, **Squeeze** the handle, **Sweep** side to side. ("A Complete Guide to PASS Fire Extinguisher Method")
- **Never use water** on electrical or flammable liquid fires.

The Fire Triangle

The **Fire Triangle** is a simple model used to understand the three essential elements required for a fire to start and sustain combustion. ("What is the Fire Triangle? - homesafetools.com") Removing any one of these elements will **prevent** or **extinguish** a fire.

The Three Elements of the Fire Triangle:

1. Heat

Definition: The energy source that raises a material to its ignition temperature.

Examples:

- Open flames (matches, lighters)
- Electrical sparks or faults
- Hot surfaces (cookers, machinery)
- Friction (mechanical grinding)
- Static electricity

Role: Heat is necessary to initiate the combustion process by raising the temperature of a fuel to its **ignition point**.

2. Fuel

Definition: Any combustible material that can burn.

Types of Fuel:

- **Solids**: Wood, paper, fabric, plastics
- **Liquids**: Petrol, paraffin, alcohol, cleaning solvents
- **Gases**: Methane, propane, butane, hydrogen
- **Role**: Fuel is the material that burns and sustains the fire once it is ignited.

3. Oxygen

Definition: The oxidising agent that supports the chemical reaction of combustion. In most fires, this is oxygen in the air.

Normal concentration in air: ~21%

Sources:

- Atmospheric oxygen
- Compressed oxygen (e.g. in medical cylinders)
- Chemical oxidisers (e.g. nitrates, chlorates)

- **Role**: Oxygen reacts with the fuel and heat to sustain the combustion process.

How the Fire Triangle Works

When all three elements — **heat, fuel,** and **oxygen** — are present in the right proportions, a chemical reaction called **combustion** occurs, resulting in fire.

▲ **Fire = Heat + Fuel + Oxygen**

If **any one element is removed**, the fire will be extinguished: ("Microsoft Word - 5327 Guide.docx - AP Safety Training")

- Remove **heat** → Use water to cool.
- Remove **fuel** → Shut off gas or isolate combustibles.
- Remove **oxygen** → Smother with foam, CO_2, or fire blanket.

Application in Firefighting

Understanding the Fire Triangle helps in selecting appropriate fire-fighting methods:

Method	Removes	Example
Cooling	Heat	Water extinguisher on Class A fire
Smothering	Oxygen	CO_2 on electrical fires, fire blanket on cooking oil
Starvation	Fuel	Turning off gas supply, removing nearby combustibles

▲ The Fire Tetrahedron (Advanced Concept)

"In more advanced fire science, a **fourth element** is added, forming the **Fire Tetrahedron:**" ("MILLARVILLE HISTORICAL SOCIETY> - Facebook")

4. Chemical Chain Reaction

Once a fire starts, **free radicals** in the flame sustain the combustion reaction. Certain extinguishing agents (like dry powder) interrupt this **chemical chain reaction**, effectively extinguishing the fire even if heat, fuel, and oxygen are still present.

Key Takeaways

- "The **Fire Triangle** is fundamental to fire prevention and response." ("Back to the Basics: Fire Triangle Fundamentals")
- **Removing one side** of the triangle will stop the fire.

- Fire risk assessments and fire safety training should always refer to the Fire Triangle model to explain ignition risks and control measures.

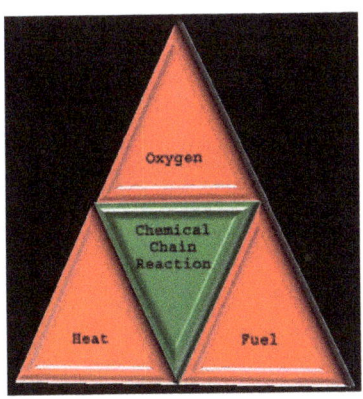

How Fire Spreads

How Fire Spreads

Understanding how fire spreads is critical for effective fire prevention, risk assessment, and emergency response. Fire spreads through **three primary mechanisms**:

1. Conduction

Definition:
Conduction is the transfer of heat through a solid material from one molecule to another, without the movement of the material itself. ("5 Types of Heat Transfer Methods in Thermal Engineering")

Key Points:

- Heat travels through materials, especially **metals**, which are excellent conductors.
- For example, heat from a fire can travel through metal pipes or structural supports and ignite flammable materials in other areas.
- **Fire doors**, insulation, and compartmentation are designed to reduce heat transfer by conduction.

2. Convection

Definition:
Convection is the transfer of heat by the **movement of hot gases or liquids**, typically rising due to being less dense.

Key Points:

- Hot air and smoke rise and spread through stairwells, corridors, and ventilation systems.
- This explains why ceilings and upper floors often experience the most heat damage.
- Convection currents can rapidly carry flames and hot gases to other areas of a building, escalating the fire risk.

3. Radiation

Definition:
Radiation is the transfer of heat in the form of **electromagnetic waves**, without requiring direct contact or a medium.

Key Points:

- Radiated heat travels in all directions from the fire, much like sunlight.
- It can ignite nearby materials even without physical contact — for example, heat from a burning vehicle can ignite an adjacent one.
- Radiation is especially dangerous in tightly packed spaces or when combustible materials are stored close together.

⟳ Summary

Method	How it Works	Example Scenario
Conduction	Heat travels through solid materials	Fire spreads through metal beams or cables
Convection	Hot gases rise and circulate	Flames move up stairwells or vents
Radiation	Heat radiates as energy waves	Nearby furniture ignites from radiant heat

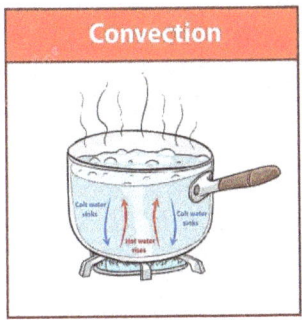
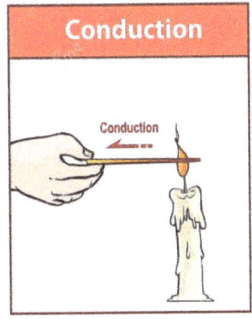
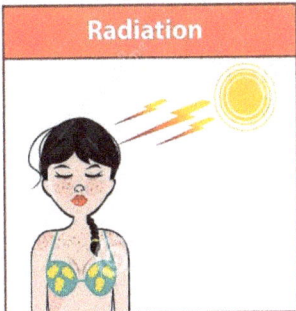

Best Fire Extinguishers for Vehicles (UK Guide)

✅ Key Requirements

When selecting a fire extinguisher for a vehicle, consider:

- **Size & weight** (space and handling)
- **Fire class coverage** (especially A, B, C, and Electrical)
- **Ease of use**
- **BS Kitemark or CE certification**
- **Corrosion-resistant materials**
- **Secure mounting bracket**

Recommended Fire Extinguisher Types

1. Dry Powder (ABC) Extinguisher

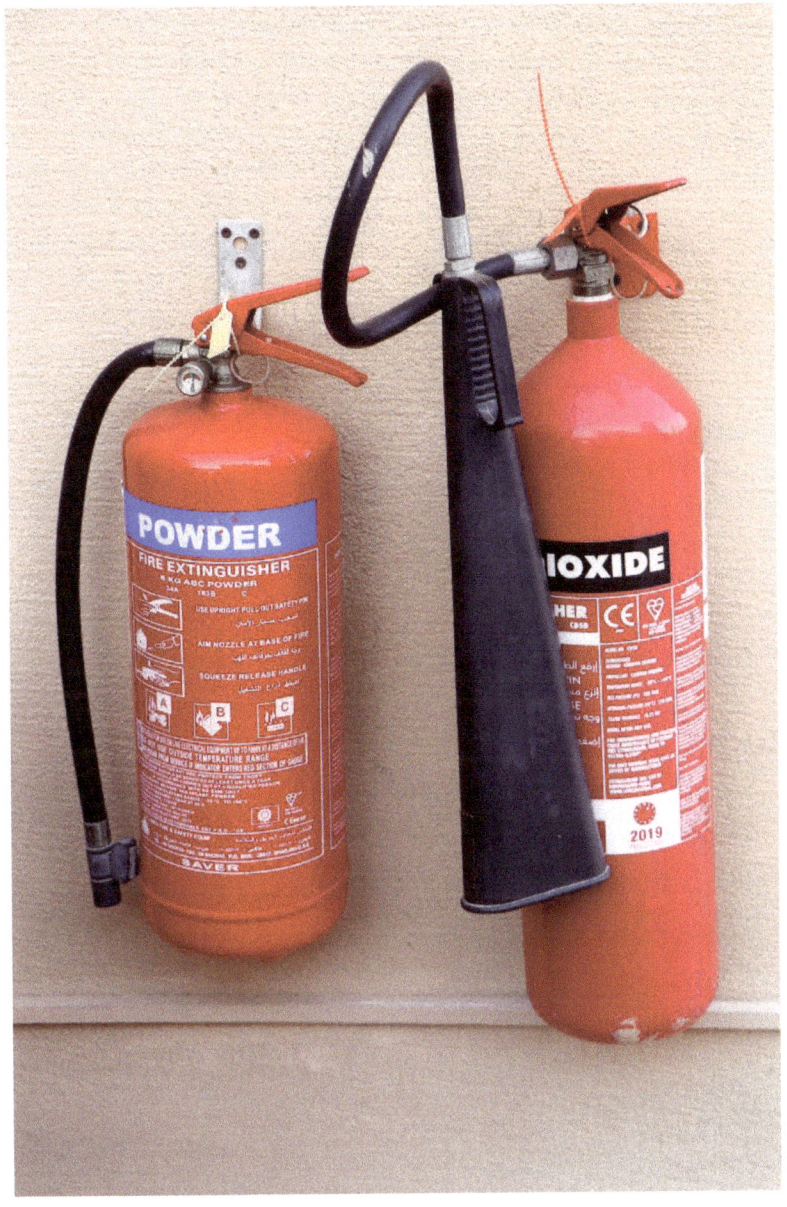

Best for: Cars, vans, 4x4s, motorbikes, caravans, motorhomes, HGVs

- **Covers Classes A, B, C and Electrical fires**
- Suitable for solid combustibles (A), flammable liquids (B), and gases (C)
- Safe on live electrical equipment
- **Compact sizes** available: 600g, 1kg, 2kg

Pros:

- Very versatile
- Fast knockdown of flames
- Compact & lightweight

Cons:

- Leaves powder residue (can damage electronics)
- Not ideal in enclosed spaces without ventilation

Recommended model:

- 1kg or 2kg **ABC dry powder extinguisher**
- Must comply with **BS EN 3**, with **pressure gauge**, mounting bracket, and **CE/UKCA marking**

2. Foam (AFFF) Extinguisher

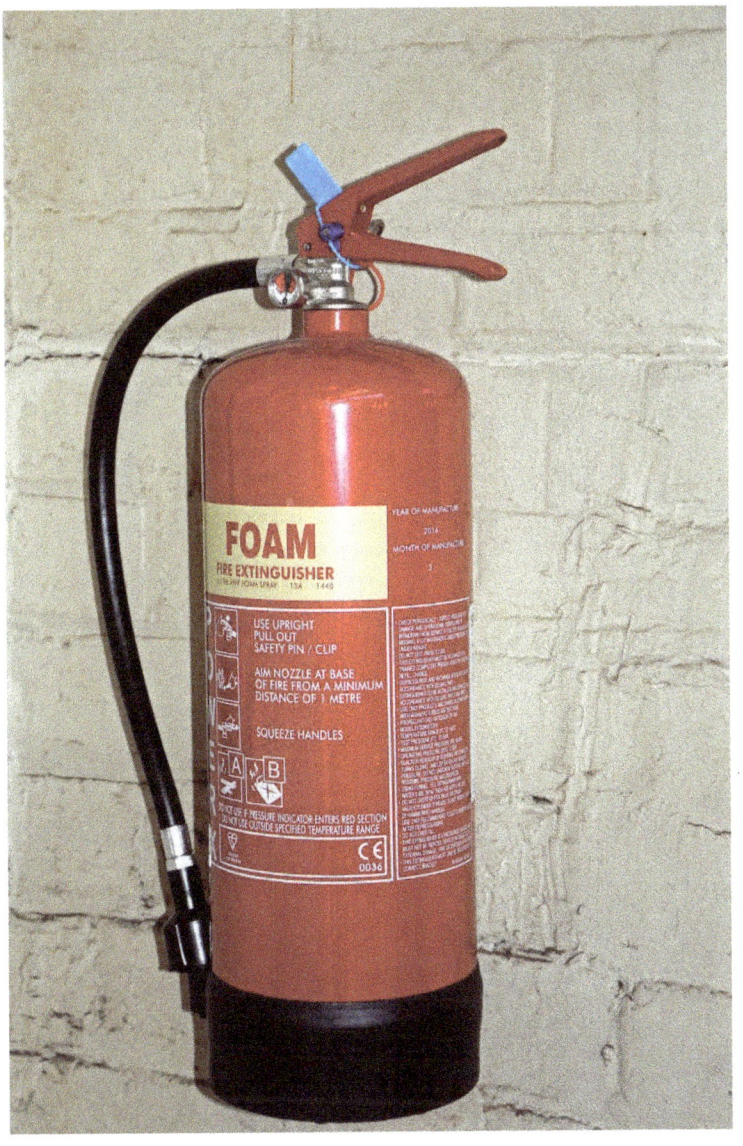

Best for: Private cars or light vehicles with emphasis on flammable liquids (petrol/diesel)

- Covers Class A and B fires
- More effective than water for flammable liquids

- Minimal cleanup compared to powder

Pros:

- Good for fuel fires
- Gentle on interiors
- Compact units (1–2 litres) available

Cons:

- Not effective on gas fires (Class C)
- **Not safe on live electrical equipment**

Use with caution: Only if electrical risks are fully isolated.

3. CO_2 (Carbon Dioxide) Extinguisher

Best for: Vehicles with sensitive electronics (e.g. EVs, luxury cars, or buses)

- Covers **electrical fires** and **flammable liquids**
- Leaves **no residue**
- Does not damage electronics

Pros:
- Ideal for dashboards and battery compartments
- Clean agent – no cleanup

Cons:
- No Class A (solid materials) coverage
- Limited cooling effect

- Not effective outdoors (gas can disperse)
- **Size**: 2kg unit minimum for vehicle use

3. Wet Chemical (Class F) Extinguisher

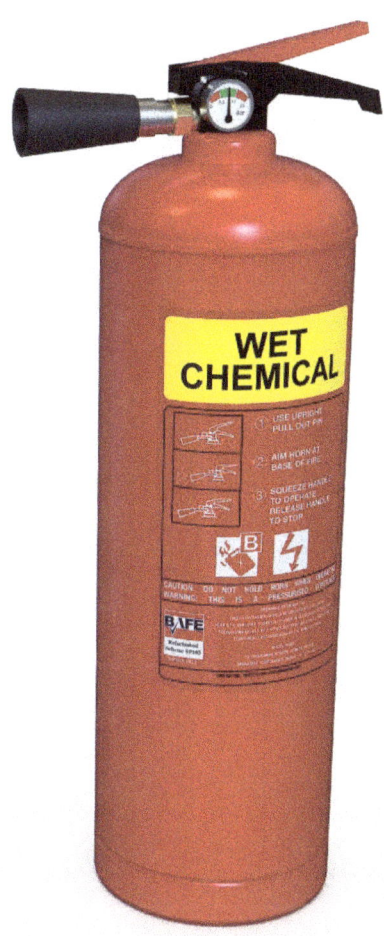

Specialists use only: **Not generally required for vehicles**, unless cooking appliances are present (e.g. food trucks, campervans)

- Designed for **cooking oil fires**
- Class F and limited A fire protection

Best Practice by Vehicle Type

Vehicle Type	Recommended Extinguisher	Suggested Size
Private Car	1kg ABC Dry Powder OR 1L Foam	1kg / 1L
Van / 4x4	2kg ABC Dry Powder	2kg
Motorhome / Camper	2kg ABC Dry Powder + Fire Blanket	2kg
Motorcycle	Small 600g–1kg ABC Powder (in soft case)	600g–1kg
Food Van	2L Wet Chemical + 2kg ABC Powder	As required
HGV / LGV	2kg–6kg ABC Powder (check operator policies)	Min 2kg
Electric Vehicle	2kg CO_2 OR 2kg ABC Powder	2kg

⚑ Additional Tips

- Always **secure extinguishers** with a **mounting bracket** (legally required for commercial vehicles).
- Regularly **check the pressure gauge** and ensure servicing per **BS 5306-3** (annually for commercial use).
- Label the extinguisher type clearly and include usage instructions.

- Consider adding a **fire blanket** for cooking or upholstery fires (especially in campers or caravans).

Fire Extinguishers

There are five main types of fire extinguishers.

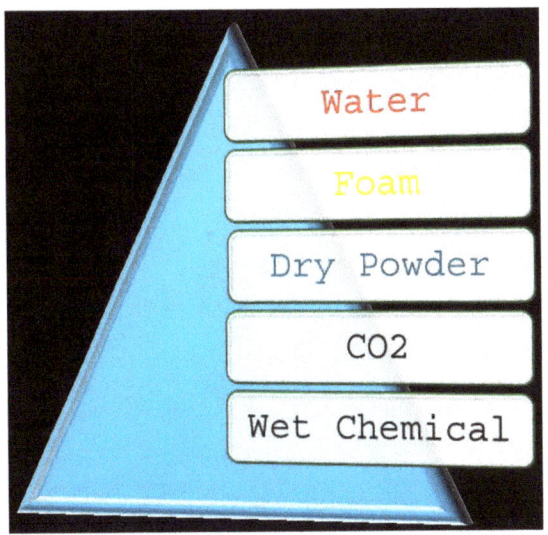

Colour Markings BS EN3

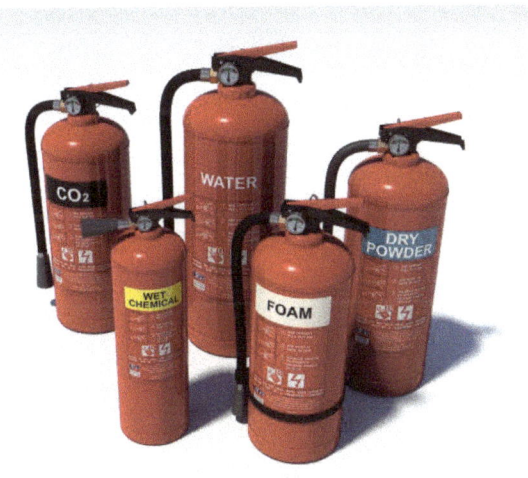

Water Extinguisher

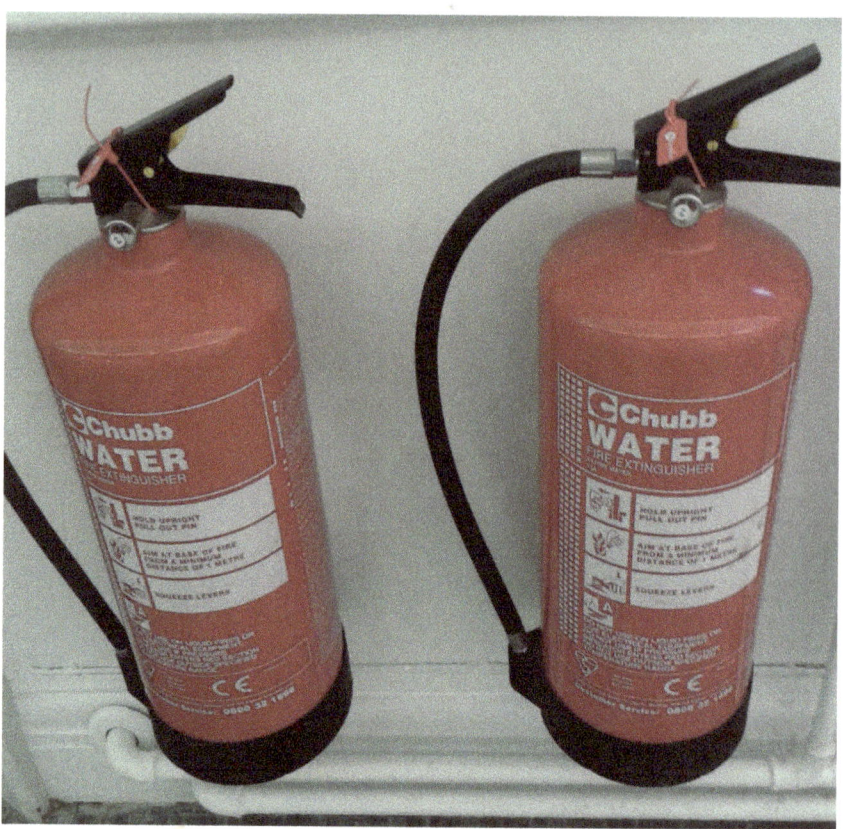

- For use on class A fires.
- Extinguishes by cooling.
- 40 – 50 seconds duration.
- IMPORTANT: Do not use fuel, electrical, or chip pan fires as it will cause a violent reaction.

Foam Extinguisher

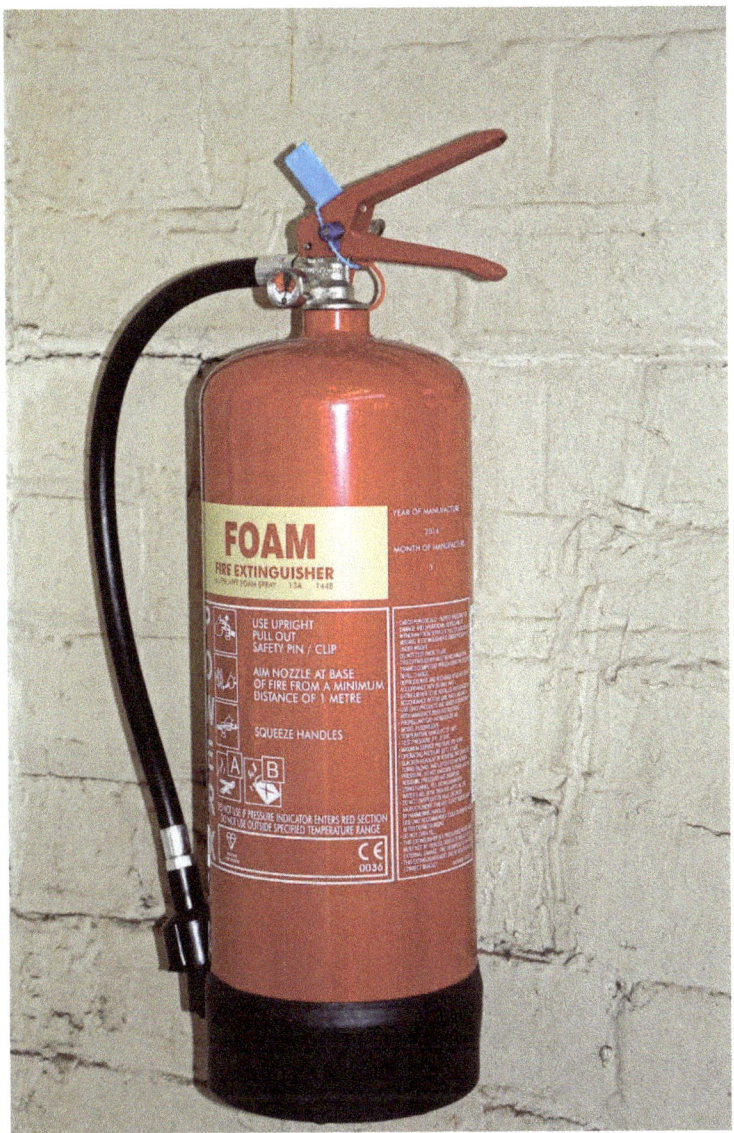

- Use on class A or B fires.
- Extinguishes by forming a blanket to inhibit the air supply.
- 35 – 40 seconds duration.

- IMPORTANT: Do not use electricity on fires as it is water-based.

Dry Powder Extinguisher

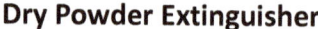

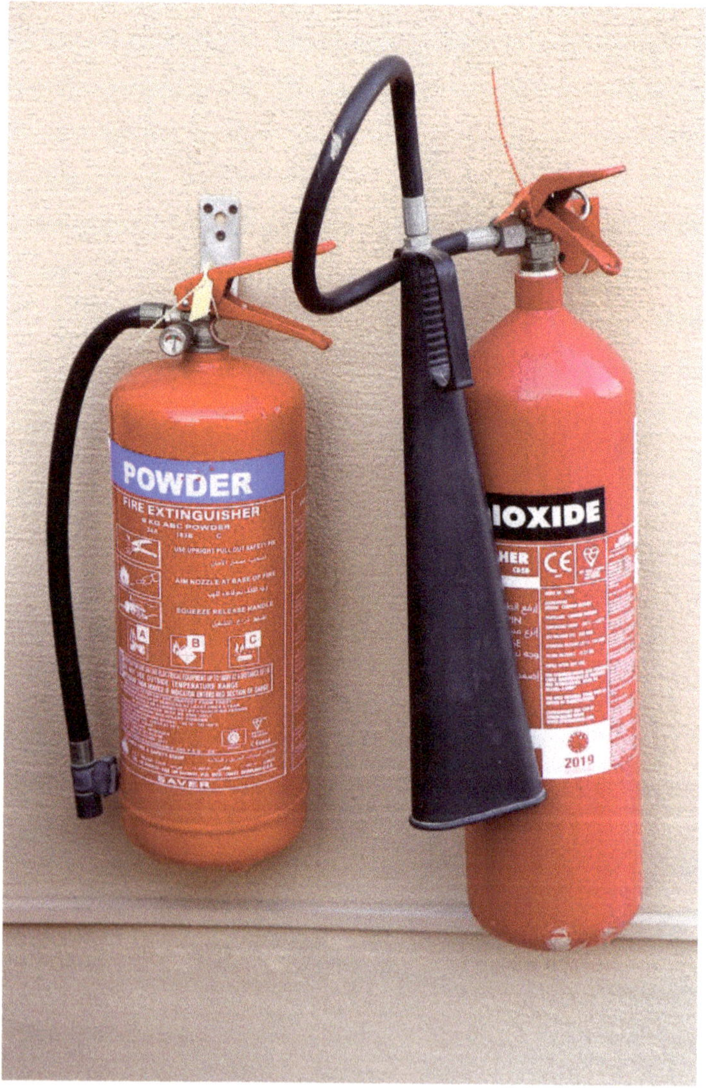

- For use in classes A + B + Electrical fires.
- Extinguishes by smothering and cooling.

- Duration depends on size.
- Particularly effective on car engine fires. (Keeping the bonnet on the latch).
- It is difficult to use in windy conditions.
- Creates a lot of mess if used indoors.

Carbon Dioxide (CO2) Fire Extinguisher

- For use on Electrical fires + class B fires.
- Extinguishes by smothering.
- Duration depends on size.
- Clean extinguishing agent that does not cause much damage.
- Danger from frost on discharge horn. Protect with a sleeve or do not touch.

Wet Chemical

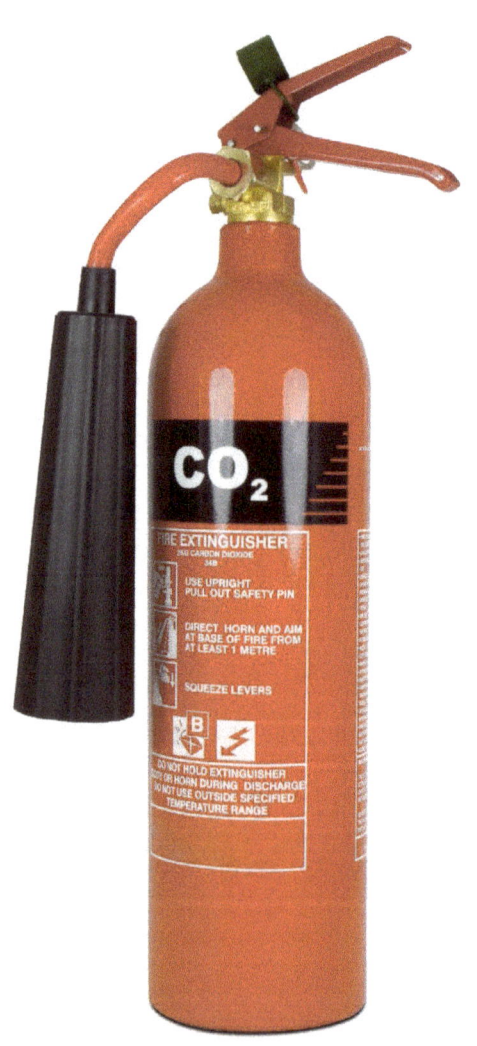

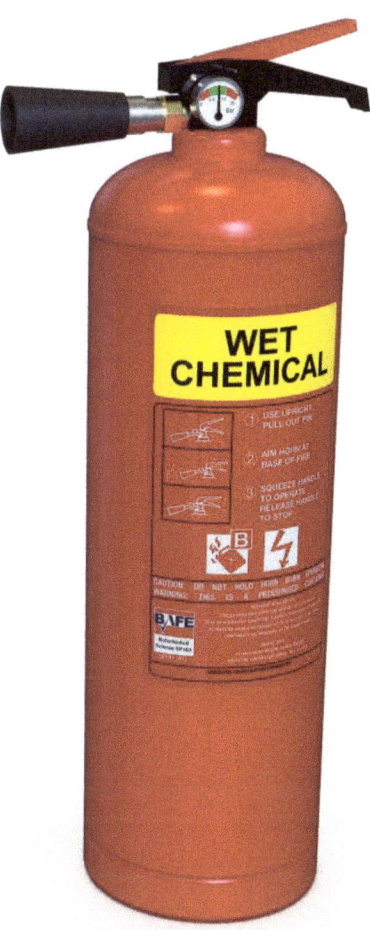

- For use on class F fires — involving cooking oils & fats. ("Types Of Fire Extinguishers - A Guide - Fire Risk Assessment Network")
- Usually recommended for kitchens.
- Extinguishes by smothering — chemical reaction seals the fire.
- Can be used on class A fires.
- 43 seconds with a 4 m jet range.

- Not to be used on electrical equipment

Electric Vehicles

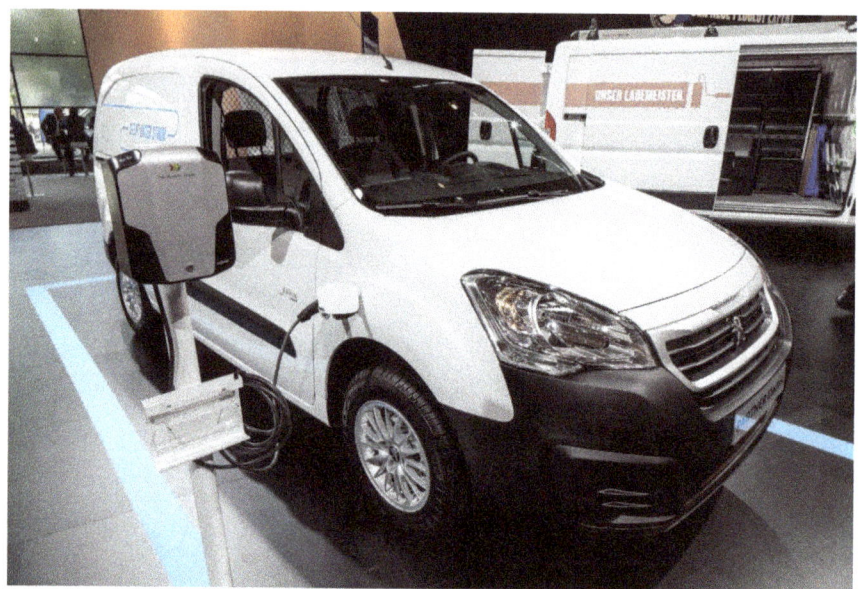

- Powered by Lithium-ion battery.
- Over one hundred organic chemicals are released when EVs catch fire, all of which are fatal to humans. Examples include carbon monoxide and hydrogen cyanide.

The best fire extinguisher for EVs is the Lith EX Fire Extinguisher.

500ml Lith-Ex Fire Extinguisher

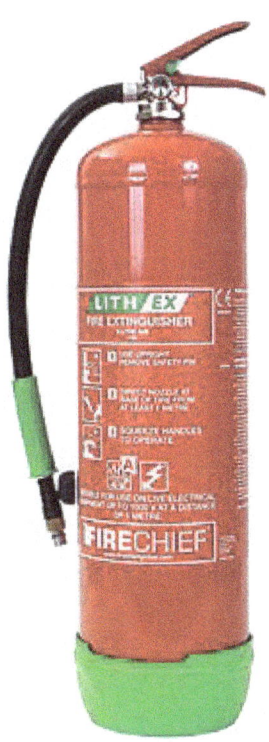

Used for fires caused by Lithium-Ion batteries.

Lithium-Ion Batteries are found in:
- Phones
- Tablets
- Laptops
- Camera
- Power tools

This fire extinguisher uses AVD (Aqueous Vermiculite Dispersion), which is a fire extinguishing agent. This creates a film over the surface of the fuel and acts as a barrier to oxygen, cools the area, and stops reignition.

An ABC fire extinguisher will not extinguish battery fires. The Lith-Ex Fire Extinguisher is suitable for class A fires and live fires of up to 35 KV.

1 KG ABC Powder Fire Extinguisher for Cars

A dry powder, category ABC fire extinguisher is most suitable for cars. ("A guide to vehicle fire extinguishers | Halfords UK")
However, they're not recommended for confined spaces and should be avoided for caravans or motor homes.

AFFF Fire Extinguishers - Suitable for Cars (Aqueous film forming foam)

Suitable for use in confined spaces

BS EN3 approves.

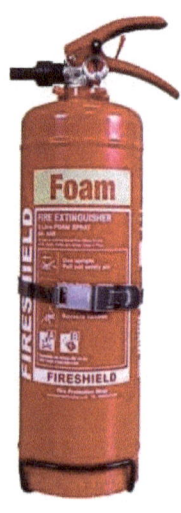

Vehicles Legally Required to Carry Fire Extinguishers (UK)

Certain vehicles operating in the UK are **legally required** to carry **appropriately sized and approved fire extinguishers** as part of their fire safety obligations. These requirements help ensure the safety of drivers, passengers, and other road users.

🔍 Legal Basis

- **The Road Vehicles (Construction and Use) Regulations 1986**
- **"The Public Service Vehicles (Conditions of Fitness, Equipment, Use and Certification) Regulations 1981"** ("File:The Public Service Vehicles (Conditions of Fitness, Equipment, Use ...")
- **Health and Safety at Work etc. Act 1974**
- **Regulatory Reform (Fire Safety) Order 2005**
- **Operator licensing regulations (e.g., DVSA and Traffic Commissioner requirements)**

✅ Vehicles That Must Carry Fire Extinguishers

🚗 Taxis

- All licensed taxis and private hire vehicles (PHVs) are typically required by **local licensing authorities** to carry at least one **approved fire extinguisher**.
- Must be **securely mounted**, accessible to the driver, and regularly inspected.

- Most councils require a **1kg dry powder** extinguisher as a minimum.

🚐 Minibuses (8–16 passengers)

- Required to carry at least **one portable fire extinguisher** suitable for **Class A, B, and C fires**.
- Must be compliant with **BS EN 3** and adequately maintained.
- Where passengers are carried, **multiple extinguishers may be required**, especially in longer vehicles.

Buses

- Must be fitted with **at least one fire extinguisher**.
- Additional extinguishers may be required based on vehicle size and passenger capacity.
- Fire extinguishers must be:
    - Easily accessible
    - Suitable for electrical and flammable liquid fires
    - Serviced regularly per **BS 5306-3**

Coaches

- Subject to similar requirements as buses.
- Fire extinguishers must be suitable for engine, passenger, and driver areas.
- A **minimum of two extinguishers** is often required:
    - One near the driver
    - One near the rear or engine bay

🚌 Public Service Vehicles (PSVs)

- All PSVs must carry fire extinguishers appropriate to the vehicle's risks.
- Must meet conditions under **Public Service Vehicle (Condition of Fitness, Equipment, Use and Certification) Regulations**.

🚚 Commercial Transport Vehicles (e.g., HGVs, LGVs)

- Requirements vary by **load type**, **vehicle classification**, and whether the vehicle carries **dangerous goods**.
- **ADR vehicles** (transporting hazardous materials) must carry:
    - At least **1x 2kg** extinguisher for the cab
    - Additional extinguishers depending on vehicle size and load type (up to 12kg total)
- Employers have a duty under the **Health and Safety at Work Act** to ensure employees driving commercial vehicles are equipped with fire safety equipment appropriate to their work environment.

General Safety & Maintenance Requirements

Fire extinguishers must:

- Conform to **BS EN 3**
- Be **securely mounted** and **readily accessible**
- Be **regularly inspected and maintained** (at least annually for commercial use)
- Have clear **instructions for use** and proper **signage**

Recommended Types of Extinguishers for Vehicles

- **1kg–2kg ABC Dry Powder** extinguisher (covers Class A, B, C & electrical)
- CO_2 extinguisher for **sensitive electronics** or passenger comfort areas
- **Wet Chemical** extinguisher in food vans or mobile catering vehicles
- Fire **blanket** (optional, but recommended in campervans, taxis, or food vehicles)

Best Practice

- Carry out **fire risk assessments** for vehicle fleets.
- Provide **driver training** on extinguisher use.
- Maintain **servicing records** for inspection by licensing or enforcement authorities.

Fire Safety Rules for Company Cars (UK Guidance)

While there is **no specific legal requirement** for standard **company cars** to carry a fire extinguisher, employers still have clear responsibilities under UK **health and safety legislation** to protect staff who drive for work purposes.

Legal Duties for Employers

Under the:

- **Health and Safety at Work etc. Act 1974**
- **Management of Health and Safety at Work Regulations 1999**

Employers are required to:

- Conduct a **suitable and sufficient risk assessment** for all work-related driving activities, including those carried out in company cars.
- Implement appropriate **control measures** to reduce any identified risks — including fire risks — as far as is reasonably practicable.

⍰ Fire Extinguishers in Company Cars

Although not legally mandatory, providing a **small, approved fire extinguisher** in company cars is considered a **best practice** safety measure, especially for:

- Staff driving long distances or in remote areas

- Vehicles carrying **technical, electrical, or flammable equipment**
- Field engineers, surveyors, or mobile workers
- Hybrid or electric vehicles (due to battery fire risk)

A typical recommendation is a **1kg ABC dry powder extinguisher**, conforming to **BS EN 3**, with a secure mounting bracket and pressure gauge.

Contractual and Local Authority Requirements

Some **local authorities**, government departments, or corporate clients may:

- Require fire extinguishers as part of their **contractual conditions** for service providers or subcontractors
- Include fire safety equipment (including extinguishers and first aid kits) in vehicle safety audits or **tender specifications**

Employers bidding for or working under such contracts should check the relevant **tender documentation** or **framework agreements** to ensure compliance.

Best Practice Recommendations

- Provide a fire extinguisher in company vehicles as a **precautionary safety measure**
- Ensure extinguishers are:
    - **Appropriate to the fire risk**
    - **Securely fitted** and regularly maintained
    - **Accompanied by basic fire awareness training**

- Include fire safety equipment in the company's **vehicle use policy**

ADR & CDG Regulations: Fire Extinguisher Requirements for Vehicles Carrying Dangerous Goods

◆ **What Is ADR?**

ADR stands for:

"Accord européen relatif au transport international des marchandises Dangereuses par Route"

(English: **European Agreement concerning the International Carriage of Dangerous Goods by Road**) ("Understanding the ADR Licence: Comprehensive Guide")

Despite Brexit, **ADR remains in force in the UK** via the **Carriage of Dangerous Goods and Use of Transportable Pressure Equipment Regulations 2009** (as amended), also referred to as the **CDG Regulations**.

Which Vehicles Must Comply?

Vehicles transporting **hazardous materials** — including chemicals, fuels, gases, or infectious substances — must comply with ADR fire safety provisions, including the **carriage and maintenance of fire extinguishers**.

ADR Fire Extinguisher Requirements by Vehicle Weight

Vehicle Type (Maximum Permissible Mass)	Minimum Fire Extinguisher Provision
Up to 3.5 tonnes	1 × 2kg + 1 × 2kg (dry powder) = 4kg total
Between 3.5 – 7.5 tonnes	1 × 2kg + 1 × 6kg = 8kg total
Over 7.5 tonnes	1 × 2kg + 1 × 6kg (or more) = 8kg+ total
Small Load Threshold or Infectious Substances Only	1 × 2kg dry powder extinguisher

🔧 **Positioning & Accessibility**

- At least one extinguisher must be **within reach of the driver's seat**
- Others should be **mounted externally or in accessible vehicle compartments**
- Fire extinguishers must be suitable for **engine and load fires**, covering **Class A, B, C**, and **electrical** risks (i.e. **ABC dry powder**)

ADR Applies to:

- Lorries, trucks, and vans carrying dangerous goods
- Vehicles transporting fuels, corrosives, flammable liquids/gases, oxidisers, toxic substances, and infectious materials

- Both **full ADR loads** and **'small load exemptions'** (though requirements differ)

Fire Extinguisher Maintenance Requirements

To comply with both ADR and CDG regulations, fire extinguishers carried on vehicles must be:

🔍 Inspected and Maintained As Follows:

- **Visual inspections** carried out **regularly** (e.g. weekly or pre-use)
- **Annual servicing** by a competent person, in line with **BS 5306-3**
- A **label or tag** indicating the **next service due date** must be attached
- Replace extinguishers if:
    - They are **damaged**, **depressurised**, or missing safety seals
    - They are **more than 10 years old**, even if unused

⚠ Non-Compliance Risks

Failure to comply with ADR fire extinguisher requirements may result in:

- **Prosecution under CDG regulations**
- **Prohibition notices** or **fines** by the DVSA or HSE
- **Insurance invalidation** in the event of an incident

Common Causes of Vehicle Fires

Vehicle fires can occur for a variety of reasons, many of which are preventable through proper maintenance, design awareness, and early fault detection. Below are the key causes:

🔧 1. Design and Manufacturing Defects

- Faulty **vehicle design**, including poorly protected fuel systems, electrical layouts, or battery placements, can lead to increased fire risk.
- **Manufacturer recalls** may sometimes be issued to address these fire hazards.

🚗 2. Road Traffic Collisions

- **High-impact accidents** can rupture fuel lines, electrical systems, or battery compartments, creating ignition sources.
- Sparks from metal-on-metal friction, combined with flammable fluids, significantly increase fire likelihood after a crash.

🛠 3. Poor Maintenance Practices

- Inadequate or irregular servicing can result in:
    - **Leaking fluids** (e.g., oil, fuel, transmission fluid)
    - **Cracked hoses** or **worn-out seals**
    - **Clogged filters** and overheating components
- Delayed attention to dashboard warning lights may also allow minor issues to escalate into fire hazards.

⚙ 4. Mechanical Failures

- Common mechanical causes include:
    - **Overheating engines** or cooling systems
    - **Broken or degraded belts and hoses**
    - **Loose or leaking fuel or oil lines**
- These components can ignite when exposed to high engine temperatures or electrical sparks.

🔌 5. Electrical System Faults

- One of the **most frequent causes** of vehicle fires.
- Risks include:
    - **Damaged or frayed wiring**
    - **Poorly installed aftermarket electrical accessories**
    - **Corroded battery terminals**
    - **Loose connections**, which may cause arcing
- Sparks from electrical faults can ignite **hydrogen gas** released by the battery or nearby combustibles.

6. Overheating Systems

- **Malfunctioning cooling systems**, low coolant levels, or broken fans can cause engines and surrounding components to overheat.
- Excessive heat in confined engine bays can ignite plastics, insulation, or spilled fluids.

7. Arson and Malicious Damage

- Vehicles may be deliberately set on fire as an act of vandalism or criminal intent.
- Arson is a **criminal offence** under the Criminal Damage Act 1971 and poses risks to surrounding property and life.

8. Failed Brake or Locking Systems

- **Brake lockups** or seized components generate excessive heat through friction.
- If combined with flammable brake fluid leaks or debris, this can start a fire in the wheel arch or undercarriage area.

Prevention Tips

- Maintain regular **vehicle servicing** and **fluid checks**
- Inspect **electrical systems** and **battery terminals**
- Respond promptly to **warning lights** and **unusual smells**
- Avoid overloading circuits with **non-standard accessories**
- Park in **secure, monitored areas** to deter arson

AFFF FIRE EXTINGUISERS

Examples of AFFF Fire Extinguishers (Previously Common in the UK)

Model Name / Brand	Capacity	Fire Classes	Notes
Fire chief AFFF Foam Extinguisher	6L / 9L	A, B	Widely used in commercial premises; contains PFAS-based foam
Chubb FX AFFF Foam	6L / 9L	A, B	Traditional model; check SDS for PFOS/PFOA content
Jactone Premium Foam (AFFF)	6L	A, B	Includes internal lining; manufacturer now offering FFF versions
Commander EDGE AFFF Foam Extinguisher	6L	A, B	High performance rating (e.g. 21A 183B); PFAS-containing
Gloria S6F Foam Extinguisher	6L	A, B	German brand common in UK; now being replaced by FFF
Thomas Glover AFFF Foam	6L / 9L	A, B	Standard in many offices and warehouses
Power X Foam (by Firemark)	6L	A, B	May contain C6 fluorochemicals – still requires replacement

Important:

- These extinguishers were compliant when released, but if they **contain long-chain PFAS like PFOA or PFOS, they must be replaced by 4 July 2025.**
- Some manufacturers now offer **fluorine-free foam (FFF) versions** of these same models — always check the product specification or SDS.

Replacement Options (Fluorine-Free / PFAS-Free)

Model / Brand	Type	Notes
Fire chief F3 Foam	Fluorine-Free	Certified for use in Class A & B fires
Jactone P50 FFF Foam Extinguisher	FFF Foam	Long-life service-free model; corrosion resistant
Commander EDGE FFF Foam	FFF Foam	Replacement for legacy AFFF models
Firexo ALL Fire Extinguisher	Multi-Class	Covers A, B, C, D, Electrical & F Fires – FFF-based
Britannia P50 Foam	FFF Foam	EN3 certified; no PFAS; 10-year lifespan

What Are AFFF Fire Extinguishers?

AFFF (Aqueous Film Forming Foam) fire extinguishers are used primarily for **Class B fires** (flammable liquids like petrol, diesel, oil, paints) and **Class A fires** (combustibles like wood, paper, and textiles).

They work by forming a **film of foam** over the fuel surface, **cooling** the fire and **cutting off oxygen**, which helps prevent re-ignition.

AFFF contains synthetic chemicals known as **PFAS** (per- and polyfluoroalkyl substances), including **PFOA** and **PFOS**, which are now linked to environmental contamination and serious health risks. These are often called "forever chemicals" because they do not break down naturally.

🚫 Current UK Guidelines on AFFF Use (as of July 2025)

⊘ Ban on PFAS-Based AFFF Fire Extinguishers

- **Effective Date: 4 July 2025**
- **What's Banned?**
  Fire extinguishers containing **PFAS substances** (especially **PFOA, PFOS**) will be **prohibited from use, storage, or sale**.
- **Reason**: These substances are **persistent, bioaccumulative, and toxic (PBT)** and contaminate soil and water.

What Is Still Allowed Until Then?

- **Existing AFFF extinguishers** that do not contain **banned PFAS (e.g., compliant C6 foams)** may be used until the ban date.
- **Training or testing use of AFFF is already restricted** – avoid discharging these extinguishers except in real emergencies.

What You Need to Do

1. Inventory Check

- Identify **all foam extinguishers** in your premises.
- Check **Safety Data Sheets (SDS)** or product labels for PFAS content.
- If unsure, consult the manufacturer or a fire safety professional.

2. Replace AFFF Extinguishers

- Switch to **fluorine-free foam extinguishers (FFF), water mist, dry powder**, or CO_2 units depending on fire risk.
- Replacement should be completed **by 4 July 2025**.

3. Dispose of AFFF Extinguishers Properly

- **Do NOT pour down drains or dispose with general waste.**
- Use a **licensed hazardous waste contractor** for safe and compliant disposal.
- Keep **disposal records** for compliance documentation.

Additional Legal Requirements

- **COSHH Regulations** (Control of Substances Hazardous to Health): You must assess and mitigate risks from hazardous chemicals like PFAS.
- **Environmental Protection Act 1990**: Illegal disposal of AFFF chemicals could result in fines or prosecution.

- **REACH Regulation (EU/UK)**: Restricts the sale and use of PFAS substances.

Summary of Key Actions for UK Users

Action	Deadline	Notes
Identify PFAS content in AFFF	ASAP	Use SDS, contact suppliers, or test professionally
Stop using AFFF for training	Immediately	Already restricted
Replace PFAS AFFF extinguishers	By 4 July 2025	Use fluorine-free alternatives
Dispose of old AFFF safely	Before July 2025	Via licensed waste handlers

Preventing Car Fires: Key Safety Measures

To reduce the risk of vehicle fires and maintain overall safety, follow these preventative steps:

- **Stay on Top of Servicing**
  Ensure your car undergoes regular servicing and passes its annual MOT. Adhering to the manufacturer's maintenance schedule helps identify and fix issues early.
- **Inspect Electrical Systems**
  Regularly check the battery, wiring, and electrical connections for signs of damage, corrosion, or wear and tear.
- **Monitor Cooling Systems**
  Keep coolant levels in check and ensure radiators, pumps,

pipes, and hoses are free from leaks or blockages to prevent overheating.

- **Watch Engine Temperature**
Be alerted to rising engine temperatures. If the car begins to overheat, stop driving immediately to prevent further damage or fire.

- **Act on Recalls Promptly**
If your vehicle is subject to a manufacturer recall, arrange repairs or replacements without delay.

- **Check Tyres Regularly**
Inspect tyres for wear, damage, or incorrect pressure, all of which can lead to overheating and fire risk.

- **Maintain a Tidy Interior**
Keep the vehicle clean and free of clutter. Loose items can obstruct ventilation or wiring, increasing fire risk.

- **Avoid Storing Flammable Items**
Do not keep flammable materials (e.g. aerosol cans, fuel, or cleaning products) inside your car.

- **Battery Maintenance**
Routinely check battery condition and ensure it is securely mounted and free from corrosion.

- **Equip with a Fire Extinguisher**
Carry a suitable in-vehicle fire extinguisher and ensure it's regularly checked and easily accessible.

How to Use a Fire Extinguisher on a Vehicle Fire

In the event of a vehicle fire, **personal safety comes first**. Only attempt to extinguish a fire if it is safe to do so and within your capabilities.

Initial Actions

1. **Stay Calm and Act Swiftly**
   - Put on your **hazard lights** and **safely pull over**.
   - **Switch off the engine** and release the bonnet using the internal control — **do not open the bonnet manually** as heat or flames may escape.
2. **Evacuate Safely**
   - Get all **occupants out of the vehicle immediately** and move to a **safe distance**.
   - Make yourself **visible to traffic** — use high-visibility clothing or wave your arms to alert others.
3. **Call for Help**
   - **Dial 999** and report the fire. If possible, ask a bystander to call while you prepare the extinguisher.

Using the Fire Extinguisher

4. **Assess the Situation**
   - Only attempt to fight the fire if it is **small**, localised (e.g. under the bonnet), and you feel confident doing so.
   - If safe, retrieve the **appropriate fire extinguisher** from the boot.

5. **Position Yourself Safely**
    - Keep your **back to a clear escape route** at all times.
    - Avoid standing directly in front of the fire or opening the bonnet fully — this may fuel the fire.
6. **Test the Extinguisher**
    - Briefly test the extinguisher away from the fire to ensure it works.
7. **Use the PASS Technique**
    - **P – Pull** the safety pin.
    - "**A – Aim** the nozzle at the **base** of the fire." ("How to Use a Fire Extinguisher - Thomas Jefferson University")
    - **S – Squeeze** the handle to release the extinguishing agent.
    - **S – Sweep** side to side to cover the fire area evenly.
8. **Discharge the Full Contents**
    - Use the **entire extinguisher**, even if the fire appears out.
9. **Monitor for Reignition**
    - Stay at a safe distance and watch for **flare-ups** until the fire service arrives.
    - If possible, have a **second person ready** to assist or take over.

⊘ When to Stop or Not Attempt to Fight the Fire

- If the **first extinguisher fails**, the fire is likely **beyond your control**.
- **Close all doors** and retreat to safety — do not re-enter the vehicle.

- **Never attempt to fight a fire** inside the cabin or involving fuel leaks.
- **If in doubt — get out and stay out.**

After the Fire

- Even if the fire is fully extinguished, **always call the fire brigade** to inspect the vehicle.
- Do not assume the fire is fully out until professionals confirm it is safe.

Legal Framework: Regulatory Reform (Fire Safety) Order 2005

Legal Framework: Regulatory Reform (Fire Safety) Order 2005 (RRFSO)

The Regulatory Reform (Fire Safety) Order 2005 is the main fire safety legislation in England and Wales. It places a legal duty on the **'responsible person'** (e.g. employer, landlord, or building owner) to ensure the safety of employees and others from fire risks.

Key Points:

- **Applies to** all non-domestic premises (e.g. workplaces, public buildings, care settings).
- Requires a **suitable and sufficient fire risk assessment**, regularly reviewed.
- Responsible person must **implement fire safety measures**, such as alarms, extinguishers, signage, escape routes, and evacuation procedures.
- Staff must receive **fire safety training**.
- **Enforced by fire and rescue authorities** with powers to issue notices or prosecute non-compliance.

Failure to comply can result in **fines, prosecution, or imprisonment**. ("Landlord Safety Certificate London EICR & Gas from £29")

Fire Safety Responsibilities of Employers

Fire Safety Responsibilities of Employers

(Under the Regulatory Reform (Fire Safety) Order 2005)

Employers have a legal duty to ensure the safety of employees and others from fire risks in the workplace. Their key responsibilities include:

1. **Conduct a Fire Risk Assessment**
   - Identify fire hazards, those at risk, and evaluate, remove, or reduce risks.
   - Keep the assessment up to date and review it regularly.
2. **Implement Fire Safety Measures**
   - Install and maintain appropriate fire detection, alarms, emergency lighting, fire doors, and extinguishers.
   - Ensure safe escape routes are clearly marked and unobstructed.
3. **Develop Emergency Plans**
   - Establish an emergency evacuation plan and communicate it clearly to all staff.
   - Ensure everyone knows what to do in the event of a fire. ("Printable Employee Fire Drill Checklist Template")
4. **Provide Fire Safety Training**
   - Train all staff in fire safety awareness and evacuation procedures.

- Appoint and train fire wardens or marshals as needed.
5. **Maintain Fire Safety Equipment**
    - Regularly inspect, test, and service fire alarms, extinguishers, and emergency lighting.
6. **Cooperate and Coordinate with Others**
    - Where premises are shared, coordinate fire safety efforts with other responsible persons.

Failure to meet these responsibilities can lead to enforcement action, including fines or prosecution.

Fire Safety Responsibilities of Employed Drivers

Daily Safety Checks

Check for:

- Fuel, oil, or coolant leaks
- Exposed or damaged wiring
- Excessive engine or brake heat
- Obstructed or blocked exhausts

Use the Vehicle as Intended

Do not:

- Overload electrical sockets (e.g., with phone chargers)
- Carry unauthorised hazardous materials
- Leave the engine running when unattended in risk-prone areas

Carry Fire Safety Equipment (When Applicable)

Ensure availability and awareness of:

- **In-vehicle fire extinguisher** (if employer requires it)
- Knowledge of **fire extinguisher use** (e.g., PASS method)
- Emergency evacuation procedures

Report Defects Promptly

Notify the employer or fleet manager immediately if:

- Smoke, strange smells, or electrical faults are noticed
- The vehicle shows signs of overheating
- A near-miss, or minor fire-related issue occurs

Follow Employer Policies

Adhere to all fire safety-related procedures as outlined in:

- Driver handbooks
- Safety inductions
- Fleet operating policies

Summary of Legal Responsibilities

Duty	Description	Relevant Law
Daily vehicle checks	Spot fire risks early	HSWA 1974, PUWER
Safe operation	Use equipment properly, avoid hazards	PUWER, Road Traffic Act 1988
Report risks	Inform management of defects/faults	MHSWR 1999
Follow training & policy	Adhere to employer's safety systems	HSWA 1974
Use equipment responsibly	Fire extinguishers, emergency kit, electronics	PUWER

Consequences of Non-Compliance

- **Fines or Prosecution** (for the driver or employer)
- **Increased risk of injury or death**
- **Invalid insurance claims**
- **Corporate liability under manslaughter laws**
- **Loss of employment or driving license**

Remember: Under UK law, employed drivers are not just operators—they are active participants in maintaining vehicle safety. Fire prevention begins with daily awareness and responsible action.

Scenario 1: Smoke from the Engine on a Motorway

You are driving a commercial van on the M25 when smoke begins to rise from the bonnet. You smell burning plastic.

What You Should Do:

1. **Pull over immediately** onto the hard shoulder or safest area.
2. **Switch off the engine** and turn on hazard lights.
3. **Exit the vehicle** quickly but calmly, using the nearest safe door (preferably on the passenger side).
4. **Move upwind and uphill** from the vehicle—stay at least 15 metres away.
5. **Call 999**, provide your location (use roadside markers or apps like What3Words).
6. **Do not open the bonnet**—exposing oxygen may intensify the fire.
7. **Use a fire extinguisher** only if:

- The fire is small and contained
- You are trained and feel safe to do so
- The fire is not under the bonnet or near the fuel tank

Scenario 2: Electrical Fire While Parked in a Depot

A battery-powered delivery vehicle starts emitting sparks and smoke while charging.

What You Should Do:

1. Activate the depot's **fire alarm or alert system**.
2. **Unplug the vehicle** only if it is safe and you are trained to do so.
3. **Evacuate the area** and direct others to leave.
4. Call **999**, inform them of the electrical fire and type of vehicle.
5. Alert the **site fire marshal** and consult the **emergency fire action plan**.

Scenario 3: Fire Caused by a Fuel Leak at a Forecourt

You notice a puddle of fuel under your vehicle at a petrol station, and a small flame starts near the rear axle.

What You Should Do:

1. Immediately **evacuate the vehicle** and warn others in the vicinity.
2. **Trigger the emergency fuel shut off** (if accessible).
3. Move everyone to a **safe distance** (over 15 metres).
4. **Do not attempt to extinguish the fire** near the fuel source unless trained.
5. Call **999** and notify station staff to activate site-specific protocols.
6. Report the incident to your manager or depot safety team.

CONSIDERATIONS BEFORE TACKLING THE FIRE

- Is it within your capability?
- Do you have the correct extinguisher?
- Test the extinguisher before you use it.
- Do you have an escape route?
- If you do not put it out with one extinguisher, get out.
- If you are in any doubt about your safety at any time, **GET OUT AND STAY OUT.**

RISK ASSESSMENT

Hazard - something that has the potential to cause harm.

Risk - A risk is the chance, high or low, of that harm occurring.

What is risk assessment?

A risk assessment is the careful examination of anything in your workplace that could cause people to suffer injury or ill health while they are at work.

Who should conduct the risk assessment?
- **You**
- **A competent person**, someone with training and experience or knowledge, someone who knows what they are assessing, but the ultimate responsibility rests on you.
- **Involve others in the process—staff.**
  Involve the person whose job you are assessing. They may know things which might not be evident to you.
  This process enables them to consider potential issues and develop solutions.
- An advantage of involving staff is that you will encourage them to think about what could go wrong and how to avoid problems. A risk assessment should be conducted. The person responsible and those assisting him are to look around for risks and fire hazards, establish how to evacuate the building, review

action plans, and identify the equipment needed to fight and prevent fire.

Purpose of Risk Assessment

- **Meet legal obligations** - to avoid fines and prosecution.
- Helps you determine whether you are doing enough to protect your workforce and others from harm.
- Reduces **occupational injuries.**
- **Moral** - no one deserves to die or get injured at work.
- **Financial** - potential cost savings, reduces insurance premiums and improves your reputation.

Preparations Before a Risk Assessment

- A tour of the workplace – A tour of the workplace is vital as part of your preparation for a risk assessment.
- Listen to the concerns of colleagues and staff. They are the ones on the ground. Listen to their suggestions.
- Consult others who are also responsible for the premises. **For fire risk assessments, there are five steps that you need to take:**

Vehicle Fire Risk Assessment Template

1. General Information

Field	Description
Vehicle Make/Model	[Enter here]
Vehicle Registration Number	[Enter here]

Field	Description
Vehicle Type	e.g. car, van, HGV, electric vehicle
Primary Use	e.g. commuting, delivery, service
Assessed By	[Name of assessor]
Assessment Date	[DD/MM/YYYY]
Review Date	[DD/MM/YYYY or every 12 months]

2. Fire Hazards

Fire Hazard	Present?	Risk Level	Controls / Notes
Flammable liquids (fuel, oils)	Yes/No	Low/Med/High	Check for leaks; secure storage and handling
Electrical systems (battery, wiring)	Yes/No	Low/Med/High	Regular inspection for damage or corrosion
Overheating (cooling system failure)	Yes/No	Low/Med/High	Check coolant levels; regular servicing
Smoking inside a vehicle	Yes/No	Low/Med/High	Strict no-smoking policy enforced
Clutter or waste inside the vehicle	Yes/No	Low/Med/High	Keep the interior clean and free of debris

Fire Hazard	Present?	Risk Level	Controls / Notes
Carrying flammable materials (e.g. aerosols, chemicals)	Yes/No	Low/Med/High	Secure, ventilated storage; MSDS available
Poorly maintained tyres	Yes/No	Low/Med/High	Routine checks for wear, pressure, and age
Use of inverters or aftermarket electrical items	Yes/No	Low/Med/High	Ensure correct fitting and fusing
The engine is left running while parked.	Yes/No	Low/Med/High	Avoid idling unless operationally necessary

3. People at Risk

Group	At Risk?	Notes
Driver	Yes/No	Always present
Passengers	Yes/No	Varies
Emergency responders	Yes/No	In the event of a fire
Bystanders/public	Yes/No	Especially in busy or enclosed areas

4. Current Fire Prevention Measures

- Annual servicing and MOT maintained
- Regular vehicle safety checks (including wiring, coolant, tyres)
- No smoking policy inside vehicles

- Fire extinguisher carried and accessible
- Training provided on safe extinguisher use
- Safe storage of flammable materials (if carried)
- Driver trained in emergency fire procedures
- Dash cam or telematics (if fitted) regularly maintained
- Recall notices are actioned immediately

5. Fire Detection & Fire-Fighting Equipment

Equipment/Control	Present?	Condition/Last Checked	Notes
Fire extinguisher (Foam/CO_2)	Yes/No	[Date]	Must be serviced annually
Fire blanket (if applicable)	Yes/No	[Date]	Optional for cooking appliances
Smoke alarm (for sleeper cabs)	Yes/No	[Date]	Required in HGV cabs with beds
First aid kit	Yes/No	[Date]	Include burn dressings if possible

6. Emergency Procedure

- Evacuate the vehicle and move all occupants to a safe distance.
- Call 999 and report the fire with the vehicle location.
- Only attempt to extinguish small fires if it is safe to do so.

- Do not open the bonnet fully if fire is suspected underneath.
- Close vehicle doors when exiting to contain the fire.
- Wait for emergency services — do not re-enter the vehicle.

7. Risk Evaluation and Recommendations

- | Overall Risk Rating: | ☐ Low ☐ Medium ☐ High |
- **Recommendations / Actions Required**

- [e.g., Replace outdated extinguisher]
- [e.g., Improve fire extinguisher training for drivers]
- [e.g., Dispose of AFFF extinguisher before July 2025]

8. Assessor Declaration

- I confirm that this fire risk assessment has been carried out by current UK guidance, and suitable controls have been identified and implemented where needed.

Assessor Name:
Signature:
Date:

APPENDICES

Appendix A: vehicle Driver Risk assessment Template

Vehicle Driver Risk Assessment Template tailored to promote **fire safety and general road safety**, suitable for both professional and private drivers. This template follows a structured approach using common UK risk assessment frameworks (based on HSE principles).

Company/Organisation (if applicable): _____

Assessor Name: _____
Date of Assessment: _____
Review Date: _____
Location/Area of Operation: _____

Hazard Identification and Risk Evaluation Table

For Vehicle Fire Safety Awareness

Hazard	Who Might Be Harmed	Existing Controls	Risk Level	Additional Controls Needed	Action By	Date Completed
Engine overheating or	Driver, passenger	Regular vehicle servicing,	M	Train driver on extinguis	Line Manage	

Hazard	Who Might Be Harmed	Existing Controls	Risk Level	Additional Controls Needed	Action By	Date Completed
electrical fire	s, road users	coolant checks, and a fire extinguisher onboard		her use; visual inspection before trips	r / Driver	
Fuel leakage or spillage	Driver, environment, fire risk	Fuel cap checks, no smoking signage, safe refuelling procedures	M	Equip vehicle with spill kit; conduct fire safety briefing	Fleet Manager	
Inadequate tyre pressure or worn tyres	Driver, passengers, road users	Routine tyre checks, pressure monitoring system	M	Include a tyre check in the pre-drive checklist	Driver	
Driver fatigue	Driver, passenger	Driving hours limit,	M	Fatigue awareness training;	Driver Supervisor	

Hazard	Who Might Be Harmed	Existing Controls	Risk Level	Additional Controls Needed	Action By	Date Completed
	s, road users	scheduled rest breaks		journey planning		
Carrying flammable materials	Driver, public	Proper storage containers, a fire extinguisher onboard	H	Provide risk-specific training; signage inside the vehicle	H&S Officer	
Poor vehicle maintenance	Driver, passengers, and public	Annual servicing, daily walk-around checks	H	Introduce a mandatory pre-drive inspection form	Fleet Manager	
Fire extinguisher not present or out of date	Driver, passengers	Advised but not routinely checked	H	Monthly extinguisher checks with an inspection log	Driver / Admin Officer	

Hazard	Who Might Be Harmed	Existing Controls	Risk Level	Additional Controls Needed	Action By	Date Completed
Mobile phone use while driving	Driver, other road users	Hands-free only policy	M	Enforce disciplinary measures for breach	Line Manager	
Adverse weather (rain, snow, fog)	Driver, road users	Driver awareness training, weather check before departure	M	Emergency kit in vehicle; winter tyres if necessary	Driver	

Risk Rating Key:

- **L = Low** – Unlikely to cause harm with existing controls
- **M = Medium** – Could cause harm; additional controls recommended
- **H = High** – Likely to cause harm; immediate action required

↻ Assessor Declaration

I confirm that the information in this risk assessment is accurate and that necessary measures will be taken to reduce risks:

Assessor Signature: _____

Date: _____

Manager/Supervisor Approval (if applicable):
_____

Date: _____

Appendix B: Fire Safety Training Record Template

This template is specifically designed for **vehicle drivers**, suitable for both individual records and company fleet documentation. It ensures compliance with training standards and promotes accountability in fire safety awareness.

🚚 Fire Safety Training Record – Vehicle Drivers

Company/Organisation (if applicable)_

Training Location: _____

Training Provider/Instructor: _____

Date of Training: _____

Next Review Date: _____

◆ Driver Information

Full Name	Employee/Driver ID	Vehicle Type	Licence Number

◆ Training Content Covered

Topic	Covered (✓)	Comments
Introduction to vehicle fire safety	✓ / ✗	
Common causes of vehicle fires	✓ / ✗	

Topic	Covered (✓)	Comments
Fire prevention measures (daily checks, safe fuelling, wiring)	✓ / ✗	
Recognition of fire warning signs	✓ / ✗	
Safe evacuation procedures	✓ / ✗	
Use of fire extinguishers (theory and demo)	✓ / ✗	
When not to fight a fire	✓ / ✗	
Reporting procedures and emergency contacts	✓ / ✗	
Legal responsibilities (Highway Code, Health & Safety)	✓ / ✗	

◆ **Training Assessment (Optional)**

Assessment Type	Completed	Score / Result	Comments
Written/Online Test	Yes / No		
Practical Demonstration	Yes / No		

◆ **Trainer's Declaration**

I certify that the individual mentioned earlier has completed fire safety training as outlined above and demonstrated adequate understanding of the content delivered.

Trainer Name: _____

Signature: _____

Date: _____

◆ **Driver's Acknowledgement**

I confirm that I have received and understood the fire safety training. I agree to apply this knowledge during vehicle operation and follow company and legal fire safety procedures.

Driver Signature: _____

Date: _____

Would you like me to generate this template in **Word**, **Excel**,

APPENDIX C: Fire Extinguisher User Guide for Vehicle Drivers

Fire Extinguisher User Guide for Vehicle Drivers

Important Warning Before Use

- **Only attempt to extinguish a fire if it is small, manageable, and safe to do so.**
- **Always ensure your safety and evacuate first if the fire is spreading or involves the engine compartment or fuel tank.**
- **Never open the bonnet if you suspect fire underneath—it can cause a sudden flare-up.**

✅ **Before Using the Fire Extinguisher**

1. **Park safely** – Pull over and turn off the engine.
2. **Engage the handbrake** – Prevent vehicle movement.
3. **Evacuate passengers** – Ensure everyone is at least 15–20 metres away, preferably upwind.
4. **Call 999** – Report the fire to emergency services.
5. **Identify the fire type** – Only proceed if it is safe and the fire is small (e.g., smoke from upholstery, wiring, or tyres—not complete engine or fuel fires).

🔧 Types of Extinguishers Suitable for Vehicles

Extinguisher Type	Colour Code	Suitable For	Not For
Dry Powder (ABC)	Blue	Electrical fires, flammable liquids, engine fires, tyres, and upholstery	Can reduce visibility in confined spaces
Foam (AFFF)	Cream	Flammable liquids like petrol and diesel	Electrical fires
CO_2 (Carbon Dioxide)	Black	Electrical fires	Not effective on upholstery or flammable solids

6. ✅ Most in-vehicle extinguishers are **dry powder (ABC)** due to versatility.

🧯 Using a Fire Extinguisher – The PASS Method

P – **Pull** the pin
A – **Aim** at the base of the fire (not the flames)
S – **Squeeze** the handle to release the extinguishing agent
S – **Sweep** from side to side across the base of the fire ("To use a fire extinguisher, remember the acronym "T-PASS": T-Twist the ...")

Tips for Effective Use

- Stand around **2–3 metres** away from the fire.
- Use short bursts to conserve the extinguishing agent.
- Watch for re-ignition – be prepared to use the extinguisher again. ("Do You Know How to Use a Fire Extinguisher? Free Access")
- Always position yourself **with an escape route behind you**.

⊘ Do NOT Attempt to Use an Extinguisher If:

- The fire is **near the fuel tank or under the bonnet**.
- The fire is **spreading quickly or producing toxic smoke**.
- You are **not trained or confident** in using the extinguisher.
- You are alone or in danger – **evacuate immediately**.

▪ After Using a Fire Extinguisher

- Report the incident to the authorities and your employer (if applicable).
- Have the extinguisher **recharged or replaced** immediately.
- Arrange a **vehicle safety inspection** before driving again.

APPENDIX D
LEGAL REFERENCE SUMMARY

Legal Reference Summary

This guide has been written in alignment with current UK legislation and best practice guidelines to ensure vehicle drivers understand their legal responsibilities regarding fire safety while operating motor vehicles. The following legal frameworks and regulatory documents are referenced throughout the guide:

◆ **1. The Road Vehicles (Construction and Use) Regulations 1986 (as amended) ("Work trucks - GOV.UK")**

- Requires vehicles to be maintained in a condition that does not present danger, including fire hazards from fuel systems, electrical wiring, or braking systems.
- Regulation 100 mandates that "a motor vehicle must not cause danger to any person due to the condition of the vehicle or its equipment."

◆ **2. The Health and Safety at Work etc. Act 1974**

- Applicable to professional drivers and employers operating fleet vehicles.
- Requires employers to ensure, so far as is reasonably practicable, the health and safety of employees and others who may be affected by their work activities, including during driving. ("Roles And Responsibilities Of Clients & Their Contractors")

- Includes responsibility for providing training, risk assessments, and appropriate fire safety equipment.

◆ **3. The Regulatory Reform (Fire Safety) Order 2005**

- Applies to vehicles used for work and transport in connection with a business or public function.
- Requires the responsible person (usually the employer or operator) to carry out fire risk assessments and ensure adequate fire precautions are in place—including provision of extinguishers and staff training.

◆ **4. The Carriage of Dangerous Goods and Use of Transportable Pressure Equipment Regulations 2009 (CDG Regulations) ("Carriage Regulations - HSE")**

- Applies when transporting flammable, hazardous, or combustible substances.
- Requires vehicles to carry appropriate fire extinguishers and comply with driver safety training requirements, especially under ADR (European Agreement concerning the International Carriage of Dangerous Goods by Road) regulations.

◆ **5. The Highway Code (Rules for Drivers and Motorcyclists)**

- Offers essential behavioural guidance related to safe stopping, responding to emergencies, vehicle maintenance, and avoiding actions that could cause fire risks (e.g., illegal storage of fuel, smoking while refuelling).

◆ 6. "The Provision and Use of Work Equipment Regulations 1998 (PUWER)" ("A Complete Guide to the Provision and Use of Work Equipment Regulations ...")

- Employers must ensure work equipment (including vehicles) is safe and properly maintained.
- Includes responsibility for ensuring that fire safety devices (e.g., extinguishers) are suitable, regularly inspected, and that users are trained in their correct use.

◆ 7. Insurance and Civil Liability Considerations

- Failure to adhere to fire safety regulations may result in **invalidated insurance claims**, **prosecution**, or **civil litigation** in the event of injury or loss due to negligence.
- Employers and fleet operators have a duty of care to protect staff and the public.

Note

This guide is intended as a practical educational tool and not as a substitute for legal advice. Drivers and employers are encouraged to consult with legal or compliance professionals to ensure full adherence to relevant legislation and to stay updated with regulatory changes.

Bibliography

1. **Health and Safety Executive (HSE).**
   Driving at work: Managing work-related road safety. HSE INDG382, 2014.
   https://www.hse.gov.uk/pubns/indg382.htm

2. **Department for Transport.**
   The Highway Code. GOV.UK, 2024 edition.
   https://www.gov.uk/highway-code

3. **UK Government Legislation.**
   The Road Vehicles (Construction and Use) Regulations 1986 (as amended). ("Work trucks - GOV.UK")
   https://www.legislation.gov.uk/uksi/1986/1078/contents/made

4. **Regulatory Reform (Fire Safety) Order 2005.**
   https://www.legislation.gov.uk/uksi/2005/1541/contents/made

5. **Health and Safety at Work etc. Act 1974.**
   https://www.legislation.gov.uk/ukpga/1974/37/contents

6. **"The Provision and Use of Work Equipment Regulations 1998 (PUWER)."** ("Providing and using work equipment safely - HSE")
   https://www.legislation.gov.uk/uksi/1998/2306/contents/made

7. **"The Carriage of Dangerous Goods and Use of Transportable Pressure Equipment Regulations 2009."** ("The Carriage of Dangerous Goods and Use of Transportable Pressure ...")
   https://www.legislation.gov.uk/uksi/2009/1348/contents/made

8. **British Standards Institution (BSI).**
   BS 5306-8:2012 – Fire extinguishing installations and equipment on premises – Part 8: Selection and positioning of portable fire extinguishers – Code of practice.
9. **Royal Society for the Prevention of Accidents (RoSPA).**
   Driving for Work: Fire Safety. RoSPA Driver Safety Resources, 2021.
   https://www.rospa.com/road-safety/advice/drivers/
10. **National Fire Chiefs Council (NFCC).**
    Vehicle Fires: Guidance for the Public and Businesses.
    https://www.nationalfirechiefs.org.uk
11. **Fire Protection Association (FPA).**
    Vehicle Fires: Causes, Prevention and Response. FPA Training Resources, 2020.
12. **DVSA (Driver and Vehicle Standards Agency).**
    Guide to Maintaining Roadworthiness: Commercial Goods and Passenger Carrying Vehicles. ("Guide to maintaining roadworthiness: commercial goods and passenger ...") 2023.
    https://www.gov.uk/government/publications/guide-to-maintaining-roadworthiness
13. **First Aid Tutors / Fairview Training Ltd.**
    Isaackson, B. *Fire Safety Manual.* UK: Fairview Training, 2023.
14. **"European Agreement concerning the International Carriage of Dangerous Goods by Road (ADR)."** ("No. 8940. EUROPEAN AGREEMENT CONCERNING THE INTERNATIONAL CARRIAGE OF ...")
    United Nations Economic Commission for Europe (UNECE), 2023 edition.

Glossary & Resources

Glossary of Key Fire Safety Terms

1. ABC Fire Extinguisher
A multi-purpose dry powder extinguisher suitable for Class A (solids), B (flammable liquids), and C (flammable gases) fires. Commonly used in vehicles due to its versatility.

2. Assembly Point
A designated safe location where people should gather after evacuating a vehicle or premises during a fire or emergency.

3. Automatic Fire Suppression System (AFSS)
A fire protection system that automatically detects and extinguishes fires without human intervention. May be installed in commercial or specialist vehicles.

4. Bonnet Fire
A fire originating under the vehicle's bonnet (hood), often due to electrical faults, overheating, or fuel leaks. Opening the bonnet during a fire is dangerous and can cause a flare-up.

5. Class A Fire
A fire involving ordinary combustible materials such as paper, wood, cloth, and upholstery.

6. Class B Fire
A fire involving flammable liquids such as petrol, diesel, or oils.

7. Class C Fire
A fire involving flammable gases such as propane or butane.

8. CO_2 Extinguisher
A type of fire extinguisher filled with carbon dioxide, effective against electrical and flammable liquid fires. Leaves no residue.

9. Combustion
The chemical process of burning, which occurs when fuel, oxygen, and heat are present — known as the fire triangle.

10. Emergency Evacuation
The rapid and safe exit from a vehicle during or after a fire to avoid harm from smoke, heat, or flames.

11. Fire Blanket
A safety device made of fire-resistant material used to smother small fires, especially those on clothing or cooking areas. Rarely used in vehicles.

12. Fire Extinguisher
A portable device used to control or extinguish small fires in emergencies. Must be suitable for the fire type and regularly checked.

13. Fire Risk Assessment
A structured process of identifying fire hazards, evaluating risks, and implementing control measures to reduce or eliminate the chance of a vehicle fire.

14. Fire Triangle
A model for understanding fire development: heat, fuel, and oxygen

are all required for a fire to start. Removing any one of these will extinguish the fire.

15. Flash Point
The lowest temperature at which a liquid can vaporise to form an ignitable mixture in air. Petrol has a low flash point, making it highly flammable.

16. Flammable Liquid
A liquid that can catch fire easily, such as petrol or diesel. Extra caution is needed when storing or refuelling.

17. Overheating
A common cause of vehicle fires, often resulting from engine faults, fluid leaks, or electrical issues.

18. PASS Technique
A method for using fire extinguishers: **Pull** the pin, **Aim** at the base of the fire, **Squeeze** the handle, and **Sweep** side to side. ("The PASS Method for Fire Extinguishers - Boston University")

19. Smoke Inhalation
Breathing in smoke, which can cause serious respiratory harm or unconsciousness. Often more dangerous than flames in vehicle fires.

20. Vehicle Fire
An unintended and uncontrolled fire involving any part of a vehicle. Can be caused by fuel leaks, electrical faults, collisions, or engine failures.

www.ingramcontent.com/pod-product-compliance
Lightning Source LLC
Chambersburg PA
CBHW051606010526
44119CB00056B/795